Women's Health and Social Change

Traditional distinctions between the experiences of Western women and men are breaking down and being reconfigured in new, more complex ways. The long-established life expectancy gap between men and women appears to be closing in many affluent societies. Many men appear to be far more 'body and health conscious' than they ever were in the past and there are perceptible changes in women's 'health behaviours', such as increases in cigarette smoking and alcohol consumption.

Taking a comprehensive and persuasive historical analysis, this book explores how social scientists and feminists have understood the relationship between women's lives and their health from the eighteenth century to the present day. Ellen Annandale argues that the old binary sex/gender differences that used to characterise men's and women's lives have not so much been supplanted as combined with diversity in late modern neoliberal economies, which profit from chronically unstable identities, with significant implications for women's health. This book takes a step forward and presents a new feminist analysis of the state of women's health.

Women's Health and Social Change will be of interest to academics and students working in sociology, women's studies, gender studies, social medicine, nursing and midwifery.

Ellen Annandale is Senior Lecturer in Sociology at the University of Leicester, UK.

Critical Studies in Health and Society
Series Editors
Simon J. Williams & Gillian Bendelow

This major new international book series takes a critical look at health in a rapidly changing social world. The series includes theoretically sophisticated and empirically informed contributions on cutting-edge issues from leading figures within the sociology of health and allied disciplines and domains. Other titles in the series include:

Contesting Psychiatry
Social movements in mental health
Nick Crossley

Men and their Health
Masculinity, social inequality and health
Alan Dolan

Lifestyle in Medicine
Gary Easthope and Emily Hansen

Medical Sociology and Old Age
Towards a sociology of health in later life
Paul Higgs and Ian Rees Jones

Emotional Labour in Health Care
The unmanged heart of nursing
Catherine Theodosius

Globalisation, Markets and Healthcare Policy
Redrawing the patient as consumer
Jonathan Tritter, Meri Koivusalo and Eeva Ollila

Written in a lively, accessible and engaging style, with many thought-provoking insights, the series will cater to a truly interdisciplinary audience of researchers, professionals, practitioners and policy makers with an interest in health and social change.

Those interested in submitting proposals for single or co-authored, edited or co-edited volumes should contact the series editors, Simon J. Williams (s.j.williams@warwick.ac.uk) and Gillian Bendelow (g.a.bendelow@sussex.ac.uk).

Women's Health and Social Change

Ellen Annandale

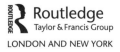 Routledge
Taylor & Francis Group

LONDON AND NEW YORK

First published 2009
by Routledge
2 Park Square, Milton Park, Abingdon, Oxon OX14 4RN

Simultaneously published in the USA and Canada
by Routledge
270 Madison Avenue, New York, NY 10016

Routledge is an imprint of the Taylor & Francis Group,
an informa business

© 2009 Ellen Annandale

Typeset in Sabon by
Florence Production Ltd, Stoodleigh, Devon
Printed and bound in Great Britain by
TJ International Ltd, Padstow, Cornwall

British Library Cataloguing in Publication Data
A catalogue record for this book is available
from the British Library

Library of Congress Cataloging in Publication Data
Annandale, Ellen.
    Women's health and social change/Ellen Annandale.
    p.cm. – (Critical studies in health and society)
    1. Women–Health and hygiene. 2. Feminist theory.
    3. Social change. I. Title. II. Series.
    [DNLM: 1. Women's Health. 2. Feminism. 3. Social Change.
    WA 309 A613w 2008] RA564.85.A56 2008
    362.1082–dc22   2008004338

ISBN 10: 0–415–19086–X (hbk)
ISBN 10: 0–415–19087–8 (pbk)
ISBN 10: 0–203–64471–9 (ebk)

ISBN 13: 978–0–415–19086–2 (hbk)
ISBN 13: 978–0–415–19087–9 (pbk)
ISBN 13: 978–0–415–64471–3 (ebk)

Contents

Acknowledgements

I began this book more years ago than I care to remember. If a positive is to be found in this, it is that since it has been so long in the writing I have had the opportunity to present aspects of it at a number of conferences, seminars and workshops. I am very grateful to those who have listened and provided constructive feedback. I would like to thank those colleagues whose shared work has influenced my thinking, particularly Judith Clark, Anne Hammarström, Kate Hunt, Ellen Kuhlmann and Elianne Riska. I am also grateful to Simon Williams and Gillian Bendelow for the opportunity to publish the book in their Series, *Critical Studies in Health and Society*, and to Grace McInnes and Eloise Cook at Routledge for their support and patience.

Introduction

We are living through a period of striking, gender-related social change in the West as traditional distinctions between the experiences of women and men are breaking down and being reconfigured in new, more complex ways. This has significant, but as yet largely unexplored, implications for health and illness. The long-established life expectancy gap between men and women appears to be closing in many affluent societies as men begin to 'catch up' with women. There are changes in the kinds of health problems that men and women suffer from, and commonsensical ideas about how men and women behave in relation to their health are in flux. Many men appear to be far more 'body and health conscious' than they ever were in the past and, while it may still be true that women 'take more care of themselves', there are perceptible changes in their so-called 'health behaviours', such as increases in cigarette smoking and alcohol consumption, which are not simply confined to the young. Pointing to changes such as these – which are, as we will see, the tip of the iceberg as far as gender and health are concerned – is not to imply that men and women are now equal or even becoming more equal in life. Nor is it to suggest that their health is converging or becoming the same. Rather, new, more complex patterns of similarity and difference, equality and inequality are emerging from the ferment. 'We literally embody the world in which we live, thereby producing population patterns of health, disease, disability, and death' (Krieger and Davey Smith 2004: 92). The question is: 'How can we understand this process?'

The theoretical stakes are high given the moral panic that gender-related social change has evoked throughout history. Conventional wisdom through recorded time has been that women and men break the social bounds and take on traditional roles and statuses of the 'opposite sex' at their peril. The currently popular view that 'liberation is a danger to women's health', for example, is widespread in media depictions of public drunkenness and other 'bad behaviours' among young women in many western nations. Although health promotion initiatives repeatedly convey the message that men's health might be improved by a reduction in stereotypically 'masculine' attitudes and behaviours, straying *too* far from 'masculine' towards 'feminine' or female-coded ways of being, in relation to health, can pose a threat to men's identities. So while changes in the experiences of women and men in the worlds of work, family, leisure and so on have been quite fast-paced of late, there remain heavy brakes on what is 'health appropriate' because health and illness still strike at the core of personal and social identity. Popular perceptions therefore rest to a large degree on how things *should* be; that is, on what is appropriate for women and what is appropriate for men. In this book, I argue that economic and cultural changes over the last thirty or so years have led to the multiple positioning of western men and women, whereby diversity has not so much replaced binary difference, but where diversity and binary difference are both in play and feed off each other. A major aim is to critically explore some of the health consequences of these changes.

The focus of the book is the health of women. This is not to imply that the health of men is not important. Indeed, there has been a surge of interest in men's health since the mid-1990s. Before then, when one saw the phrase 'gender and health' it usually meant women's health. The gendered nature of men's experience was largely invisible and hidden by assumptions of privilege. However, patriarchy, once the scourge only of women's health, is now identified as the source of many health problems experienced by men (see, for example, Lohan 2007; Riska 2004; Stanistreet *et al.* 2005). This interest in men's health is not only valuable in its own right, but also because it permits the comparative research on males and females that has been lacking until very recently. This comparative focus has been further stimulated by the adoption of 'gender mainstreaming' or 'gender sensitive' policies for health care by many governments and international agencies since the 1990s (Annandale *et al.* 2007; Doyal 2006; Khoury and Weisman 2002). This said, it is troubling and somewhat ironic that 'men's health' appears to have gained both the academic and policy spotlight as feminist interest in 'women's health' has dimmed, at least with respect to western women. This is in good part why women are the focus here. Of course, a consideration of women will involve reference to men throughout the book, not least because it is the social relations of gender as they are manifest in everyday life and framed theoretically that are the key to understanding health. But the wide-scale changes in women's lives over recent years and their impacts upon health deserve their own specific attention at the present time.

Historically, the major challenge to normative conceptions about health and the body has come from feminism. Indeed, as will be discussed in the chapters to come, health has been a crucial vehicle for the development of feminist theory dating back to at least the eighteenth century. This is as it should be. As Ellen Lewin and Virginia Olesen explained more than twenty years ago, an examination of health 'permits the revelation of those elements of western cultures which bear most directly on the construction of gender and its consequences for women, men, and the larger social order' (1985: 19). They remark that, while other domains – such as religion or the law – provide insights, none takes us as far as health does, precisely because health is so all encompassing. Yet present-day feminism has relatively little to do with health and illness. This statement may seem surprising, particularly given the recent 'corporeal' turn' (or, more accurately, *re*turn) in feminism. There is a wealth of excellent work on topics such as the body, genetics and new health technologies. Important health-related issues such as weight, eating disorders, depression related to body hatred and the difficulties of negotiating 'safe sex' have been well researched (e.g. Aapola *et al.* 2005; Brook 1999; Frost 2001; Whelehan 2000), especially where young women are concerned. But there is a general failure to attach these concerns to the material body in health and illness, that is, to address flesh-and-blood matters. More often than not, either attention stops at the body's surface or it is highly reductive in its approach to the body's interior (Birke 1999, 2003; Davis 2007a). The material body of the 'whole woman' in health and illness has receded from view.

As Ellen Kuhlmann and Birgit Babitsch (2002) aptly remark, the fault lines between feminist theory and health and illness are particularly stark. It is common enough to refer to developing theory 'through the body' (e.g. Braidotti 2002; Butler 2004; Ebert 1993; Grosz 1994), but the body in question is rarely anchored in vital matters of life and death. As others have pointed out, fears of biological essentialism led many feminists to take flight from the body from the late 1980s. These cutting and also rather amusing remarks from John Wiltshire in reference to the work of Julia Kristeva, are highly apposite:

> In this feminism, mortality is suspended – that is part of its exhilarating quality, no doubt: the implied female subject in such writing is young, bold and free, menstruates regularly and without discomfort, never suffers from lower back pain or ulcers, and not even her reading of Derrida and Lacan can give her a headache.
>
> (Wiltshire 1997: 16)

The cracks between feminism and health are equally clear in recent empirical stock-taking on the position of western women, where education, work, the family, sexuality, body image, identity and political representation all figure highly but health fails to get more than a passing mention, if that (see Bradley 2007; Charles 2002; Delamont 2001; Hughes 2002; Marshall 1994; to cite only a few). A premise of this book is that, since changes in health are a barometer of society, then feminist analysis is seriously impoverished by neglect of them. While others have argued the point that a truly embodied feminism must take account of health (see Davis 2007a; Kuhlmann and Babitsch 2002), the development of a framework to take analysis forward is still needed. In the chapters that follow I argue that health is an important vehicle for feminists to demonstrate the ways in which the lives of contemporary western women are entangled in a social economy that seemingly offers endless (liberatory) possibilities, but actually positions them in complex and contradictory ways that do not always benefit their health. It is important to make clear at this point that the book is not intended to be a detailed chronicle of empirical changes in women's lives and in their health status over time. Rather, the focus is upon *how social scientists and feminists have sought to understand the relationship between women's lives and their health*. The principal object therefore is theory development, and to this end, it is selective of particular key issues and junctures in time rather than comprehensive and attentive to all aspects of women's lives and their health. Moreover, the focus is narrowed to women in western societies, with most attention given to Britain and the United States.

The development of a framework to analyse the contemporary social relations of gender and women's health inevitably grapples with a highly charged theoretical past in relation to feminism. Given the heavy traces of early feminism in current debates, it would be unwise simply to consign 'old ideas' to history and seek to start afresh. Early feminists are often portrayed as patriarchy's imitators who, by prioritising mind over matter and reason over emotion, lacked the conceptual wherewithal to mount an effective challenge to the dualistic suppositions that sustained women's oppression. While they could hardly be expected to have stepped outside the prevailing liberal individualism, which was almost bound to direct most of their attention towards women's equal rights with men in the public spheres of employment and education, it is wrong to deduce from this that they cast health and the body aside. In fact, I wish to argue that it was quite the opposite. From the late seventeenth century through to the late eighteenth century writers such as Mary Astell and Mary Wollstonecraft not only stressed that women's oppression was socially rather than biologically caused but did so in the name of health and body politics. For this reason, we begin in Chapter 1 by travelling back in time to uncover the rich and relatively unexplored seam of women's writing on health and the body from the seventeenth century through to the early twentieth century.

The binary divisions between the social and the biological, mind and body, reason and emotion that emerged in seventeenth-century Europe made it possible to associate men with all that was valued (the social, mind, reason, action) and women with all that was generally devalued (biology, the body, emotion, passivity). By the eighteenth century, Jean-Jacques Rousseau was able to equate women with nature, and to position them as a potential source of disorder to be tamed by reason. Women, he famously wrote, can never escape their sex (or biology): 'the male is only a male now and then, the female is always a female, or at least all of her youth; everything reminds her of her sex' (Rousseau 1966 [1762]: 324). Women's unruly reproductive functions made them highly *un*qualified for public life and for occupations valued by men, such as that of physician – one shudders to think of the mistakes they would make, wrote one physician, 'at the period when their entire system, both physical and mental is, so to speak, unstrung' (quoted in Ehrenreich and English 1978: 112). But women were uniquely *qualified* for the role of patient. The sickly women of the bourgeoisie became a 'natural caste' for the emerging medical profession during the 1700s and 1800s.

During the nineteenth century, in particular, health and illness was a sensitive political barometer of socially troublesome gender identities, which feminists were able to press into the service of challenging the dualisms that nourished patriarchy. Since political commentary was not a viable outlet for most, 'health fiction' and personal narratives were a respectable way for women to raise their concerns. By conceptualising illness as a social pathology; that is, as arising out of the circumstances of women's lives (not their individual selves), many novelists, such as George Eliot and Charlotte Brontë, were able to counter the negative associations between illness and women's biology. Early women sociologists such as Harriet Martineau and Charlotte Perkins Gilman – the neglected contemporaries of the so-called 'founding fathers' – played an important role in this. We will see in Chapter 1 that they drew upon their own experience of illness and social oppression to set the seeds for an embodied sociology that was consigned to the wastelands of sociological history as the new discipline developed in a 'dys-embodied' manner due to the dominance of the agenda by the 'founding fathers', such as Karl Marx, Émile Durkheim and Herbert Spencer.

The early to mid-twentieth century is often characterised as feminism's 'silent years' (Banks 1981). But this was only a silence in relative terms. The fires that fuelled the campaigns for political emancipation may have died down (at least in a number of Western nations), but the embers were smouldering and new sparks were kindled in what became known as the 'equality versus difference' debate, as feminists contested whether women should continue to push for equal rights with men or, as the 'new' or 'welfare feminists' maintained, for protective legislation for women. It was not too long before feminists were pitched head-on into the burning disputes of the 1960s as the women's movement made health a focal concern. The 1970s were also auspicious for the difficult coming together of feminism and sociology around matters of health and illness. Chapter 2 reflects back on the unprecedented and exhilarating changes of the 'women's health movement'. The wealth of experiential data that emerged from the grass roots of the movement highlighted two crucial things: the negative consequences of male medical control of the female body and, most importantly, the ability of women to seize this control in their own interests (see, for example, Dreifus 1978; Morgen 2002).

Since patriarchy has depended on equating women with their (defective) biology, it has made perfect sense for feminists to counter with two claims:

first, that women are no more (or less) determined by their biology than are men; and, second, that the image of women's biology that patriarchy presents to the world is grossly misconstrued. These two claims unite in the proposition that women's oppression is socially caused, rather than biologically given. The basis for this argument is the distinction between biological (sex) and social (gender). Although the foundations for this distinction were laid several centuries earlier, they were built upon and taken to new conceptual heights by 'second wave' feminists from the 1970s on. The sociology of health and illness, which was developing as a new research field around the same time, also promoted the biological/social distinction. It served a political purpose here, too, enabling sociologists to claim the social as their own particular domain, distinct from biology or the biological body, which was the province of medicine.

In Chapter 2 we will see that sociological research on women's health and medicine emerged from the heady brew of barriers, breakthroughs and tensions in the relationships between the new academic feminism and activism outside the academy, and between academic feminism and wider sociology. The most pressing problem for those women who established the field was the yawning gap between their experiences as women and the theoretical frameworks that sociology (and the wider social sciences) provided to explain them. Since existing theory was incapable of accommodating feminist analysis, it had to be changed. Instituting this change proved to be both arduous and fractious and continues to the present day. The initial steps involved criticism of existing theories and extending the sociological agenda by 'adding in' the new topic of gender and, most importantly, the topic of gender *and* health. Important though these first two steps were, research was largely directed at, and limited to, reworking existing theories to accommodate women, rather than radically overturning them to develop a sociology of health that could speak for women.

Chapters 3 and 4 show that the biological (sex)/social (gender) distinction has been a conceptual treasure trove, stimulating influential and wide-ranging research on women's health and beyond. For example, studies of health status have sought to demonstrate that women's self-perceived health is generally worse than men's and that this is due to their disadvantage in access to economic and social resources, especially as they relate to employment and family life. In other words, these inequalities are socially created, not biologically given. At the same time, politically explosive research on reproductive health has drawn attention to the negative repercussions for women's health care of sexist assumptions about their bodies held by medical practitioners, especially gynaecologists and obstetricians. Many feminists working in this area during the 1960s and 1970s turned male biological privilege on its head and sought to value women's biology not only *because* it was different from men's, but because they believed it to be more powerful.

By the early 1980s, both theoretically and empirically, research was developing in two rather separate directions, which, by and large, remains the case today. On the one hand, research on gender inequalities in health has stressed parity with men, played down biological difference *from* men in favour of social similarity *to* men, and viewed the route to good health in women's equal access to positively valued social positions that traditionally have been the preserve of men. Although biology has not been cut out of the debate entirely, the main concern has been to show that women's higher levels of morbidity (illness) are *socially* created and therefore changeable. On the other hand, and far less accepted within the academy, at least in the early days, was radical feminist-inspired research, which took the reproductive body as the major site of women's oppression, and saw the route to women's emancipation in 'positive' female biological and social difference. During the 1970s and 1980s a new generation of female sociologists took this emphasis on the reproductive body and, for the first time, brought the association of health and gender to the heart of sociological analysis. As we will see in Chapter 4, the reproductive body was – and remains – more than just a new topic to be 'added in' to the existing agenda. Conceptualised as the pre-eminent – and often vexed – juncture around which women's lives pivoted, it became a rallying point for the critical, though not uncontroversial, step of challenging existing theory and developing a new theoretical understanding of the social relations of gender.

Notwithstanding these distinctions between feminists and the topics they focused on, the crucial point is that their use of the social (gender)/biology (sex) distinction led to a focus on the social and biological *differences* between men and women. This made perfect sense during the 1960s and 1970s when differences between males and females were a palpable feature of society. But it is a questionable basis for the analysis of women's circumstances and their health in the twenty-first century. By the late 1980s, research was becoming trapped in the ideological context of what it was trying to analyse, as assumptions were often made at the research planning stage about what aspects of experience were relevant for men's and for women's health, and research findings were read through the lens of this difference (Macintyre *et al.* 1996). This binary logic drew health and illness towards opposition, with the consequence that health became associated with men and illness with women. Rather ironically, it became difficult to see women as well and men as ill (Annandale and Clark 1996). Concerns about social essentialism were matched, if not exceeded, by anxieties within feminism about biological essentialism, as women's biological difference *from* men and their similarity *to* each other took precedence over those characteristics that could divide them (such as age, social class, ethnicity), and possible similarities with men were silenced. Moreover, while feminist research on health gave far more attention to embodied experience than social science generally before the advent of the 'sociology of the body' in the early 1990s, the sex/gender distinction still fostered an undue separation between the social and the biological. It is only relatively recently that researchers have come to appreciate that it may be their *interaction* that matters most in the production of health and illness (e.g. Bird and Rieker 2008; Krieger 2003; Payne 2006).

So the feminist challenge to the equation of women with their (defective) bodies through the tool of the sex/gender distinction began to look outmoded. This is not to say that the concepts of sex and gender are in themselves no longer useful – as Harriet Bradley (2007: 21) has recently put it, the 'distinction remains a vital instrument for explaining the construction of difference' – but rather that it is the binary connotations that flow from them that seem problematic. In Chapter 5, I argue that theory built on distinction is of doubtful use in much of the western world where the social relations of gender are ever more complex and fast changing, and aspects of our biology are perceived as modifiable rather than annexed in any simple way to male and female. This said, we need to be alert to the dangers in the arguments advanced by many feminists sympathetic to post-modernism – the large majority of whom write outside the context of health – that the problems arising from the 'difference approach' can be resolved by re-casting *both* social (gender) *and* biological (sex) as malleable and multiple. Certainly recent gender-related social changes in the spheres of employment, family life and leisure are releasing many women (and men) from the shackles of the past. Moreover, new approaches to biology conceptualise the 'biological body' in processual rather than fixed terms and draw attention to the development of the organism in interaction with the social world, rather than out of some blueprint in the DNA (Birke 1999; Fausto-Sterling 2005; Grosz 1994). But this does not mean that the body can be remade at will, or that the way we live our lives, and the state of our health, simply come down to free choice or individual 'life-style'. Nor, as noted earlier, does it mean that men and women are 'now equal'. Rather, the old shackles have been replaced with slippery silken ties that nonetheless bind. The nature of these ties is the focus of Chapters 6 and 7.

Chapter 6 begins by noting in general terms the complex and intertwined social changes that have been taking place in women's lives in affluent societies – in areas such as education and employment, the family and parenting, and in wider social attitudes about what is 'appropriate' for women – since the last quarter of the twentieth century. I argue that binary sex/gender differences have not so much been supplanted as combined with diversity in late modern neo-liberal economies, which profit from chronically unstable identities. I explore this though the theoretical optic of the shift from what I call an 'old single system' of patriarchal capitalism to a 'new single system'. The 'old single system' of industrial capitalism relied upon the relatively fixed and seemingly natural binary differences between men and women explored in previous chapters. But this no longer makes sense in an economy that thrives on diversity. Not only traditional 'gender roles' and statuses ('the social'), but also distinctions between sexed (or 'biological') bodies are diminishing through what Rosemary Hennessy (2000) dubs the continual tooling and re-tooling of the desirous subject. I explore the promotion of sex/gender isomorphism in product marketing, as features that might once have been considered natural, such as one's sex or 'race', have acquired the 'mutability of culture' (Lury 2002). In the 'new single system', destabilised sex/gender identities have become an indispensable condition for the cross-marketing of products and lifestyles that were once readily identified with either men or women with dubious benefits for health. It is argued that the rigid orthodoxies of the past are indeed breaking down, but they are being reconfigured in new, more complex ways, with implications for health. These changes are systemic in form, but this does not mean to say that individuals are mere dupes, pushed and pulled by a late capitalist economy that is beyond their comprehension. Juxtapositions of difference and diversity generate liberatory as well as oppressive life spaces. These spaces can never be pristine and sharply bounded. Rather, they are inescapably muddied and conflicted. It is women's lived experience within these spaces that requires our attention in relation to their health.

Chapter 7 considers changes in mortality and morbidity over the last thirty or so years. Rather ironically, it would appear that, in terms of life expectancy at least, the relatively fixed binary differences of early- to mid-twentieth-century industrial capitalism in some senses protected girls and women by keeping them away from the dangers to life and limb that cut male lives short, such as dangerous employment, motor vehicle mortality, and the risks of cigarette smoking and heavy alcohol consumption. We will see that the 100 or so years from the 1880s to the 1970s were characterised by what now appears to have been a distinct period of gradually increasing female 'longevity advantage' in much of the West. This 'advantage' began to be chipped away from the last quarter of the twentieth century onwards. Overall, life expectancy continues to grow for males and females, but the gap between them seems to be very slowly diminishing. There is also some indication that health differences during men's and women's lifetimes may either be reducing or be smaller than once thought. These changes appear to be due to both improvements in the health of men and deteriorations in at least some aspects of the health of women.

This poses a series of difficult questions. The foremost of these questions is this: if recent social change is not unequivocally beneficial for women's health, then surely this is support for the popularly conceived view that 'liberation is a danger to women's health', referred to earlier? Moreover, it would seem to vindicate long-held assumptions about women's inferiority and to throw more than 300 years of feminist analysis into doubt. It will be argued that concerns such as these are misplaced since they rely upon a highly individualised and hence 'victim-blaming' approach to health. They draw attention away from the complex interplay between individuals and social environments that has been central to feminist theorising historically.

As feminists have debated through time, age is a crucial factor in relation to women's experience and their health. First of all, since circumstances in early life impact on health later on, an individual's life course is important. Second, since people born around the same time are subject to similar social environments and lifestyle influences, age cohorts are also significant. The lives of young people are a dominant metaphor for social change, and young women in particular have become the touchstone for societal problems (McRobbie 2000). This makes the stakes unduly high in relation to moral panic around their health. Chapter 7 addresses provocative 'new feminist' writing that argues that the balance of power has altered so dramatically that we can no longer talk of patterns of male advantage and female disadvantage. It has been argued that this offers a markedly individualistic kind of radicalism where the way forward for women is lifestyle choice and self-determination (Skeggs 1997; Whelehan 2000). Yet this 'new radicalism' cannot be simply turned aside. As Stephanie Genz discusses for women generally, hybridity is the reality of many women's lives as they 'buy into standardized femininities while also seeking to resignify their meanings' (2006: 338). Although there are dangers, such as an assertiveness that ultimately is reliant on feminine allure (Whelehan 2000), there is appeal in the argument that 'gender inequality' has become a 'collective problem with an individual solution' (Aschenbrand 2006; Budgeon 2001). Women's use of different dimensions of agency slip between 'feminised agency and patriarchal recuperation' (Genz 2006: 346) and this has as yet largely unexplored implications for their health.

There have been enormous changes in women's health over the last 200 or so years. We owe our ability to interpret the state of women's health in relation to the circumstances of their lives to the groundbreaking work of feminists at least as far back as the late seventeenth century. But the worth of the theoretical tools that they bequeathed – most notably the distinction between biological (sex) and (social) gender – is increasingly in doubt. Binary difference has been combined with diversity in 'late modern' neo-liberal economies, which profit from chronically unstable identities, of which 'gender identities' are paramount. A new social tapestry is being woven whereby (biological) sex and (social) gender depend on each other for understanding just as much as before, but where the meaning and lived experience of biological sex and of social gender, as well as the connections between them, are far more fluid.

As emphasised throughout the book, this does not mean to say that women and men are now more equal, or becoming more equal, but rather that far more complex patterns of equality and inequality are arising and

– most crucially – they are written not only *on* the body, but *into* the body in new experiences of health and illness. The overall message is that, if the old theoretical tools are losing their worth, then new ones need to be forged. The chapter concludes by drawing together the key points from the earlier chapters in order to sketch in outline form what an adequate feminist analysis of women's health might look like.

1   Recovering gender and health in history

Introduction

Historian Edward Shorter (1982: xi) maintains that women were ravaged by ill health between 1600 and 1900 and that, as long as they were vastly more enervated than men, any conception of personal autonomy was meaningless. He suggests that feminism depended on – effectively waited for – improvements in women's health. Certainly women died at younger ages than men over much of this period, and living in ill health could have dampened political activity. Far more controversial is Shorter's insistence that it was the combination of the rise of (male dominated) modern medicine and new ties of sentiment between men and women that delivered women from superstition by dissolving the need for a women's healing culture and, in the process, improved their health and made feminist politics possible. In other words, ultimately it was men who were important for the development of feminism. An alternative explanation of the association between health and the rise of feminism emphasises the potential of male ideologies and practices to restrain rather than to liberate women. Throughout history patriarchal ideology has construed women's illness as inherent biological weakness. Moreover, it has been bourgeois women – the women most often in the position to pose a feminist threat – who have needed to be told that they would become ill if they ventured outside of the conventional female role. Catch 22, then: 'one way or another, by remaining in the female role or attempting to get out of it, the demon disease would attack' (Duffin 1978: 31). It is reasonable to suppose that in such a climate many women might have thought twice before risking their personal health and well-being by demanding political and social rights. But an analysis of women's writing and actions in the pursuit of health reveals that, across history, many have done exactly that: that is, both in sickness and in health, they have been far from passive subjects awaiting the enlightenment of men.

Dichotomies such as reason/emotion, mind/body and man/woman are much more than innocent contrasts (Prokhovnik 1999). Rather, they represent deep-seated polarities within Western philosophy. Heralding the new scientific age, the proposition put forward by Descartes (1596–1650) that the mind is wholly distinct from the world of matter overturned pre-modern holistic conceptualisations where illness was conceived as disharmony between the patient and their social world, and inaugurated the mechanistic conception of the body that was to underpin 'modern medicine'. Descartes' philosophy is founded on an alignment between the bodily and non-rational, distinguishing corporeal from intellectual matters (Lloyd 1993). The mind, he asserted, is entirely distinct from the body and would not fail to be what it is even if the body did not exist – hence his dictum *'cogito ergo sum'* (I think therefore I am). Existing contrasts between men and women were extended to stark polarisations as a by-product of the distinction between reason and its opposites. Qualitatively different from everyday practical thought, reason concerned 'a highly rarefied exercise of intellect, a complete transcendence of the sensuous' (ibid.: 46). In principle, this purely intellectual activity was open to all, but in reality the lives of most women meant it was hardly an option for them. Women became associated with the irrational body and men with the rational mind. Expressed as hierarchical power relations, mind–body dualism and all that accompanied it sanctioned patriarchy by permitting men to associate themselves with the positive and socially valued (the rational–mind–reason–health) and women with the negative and devalued (the irrational–body–emotion–illness).

It is widely maintained that the legacy of philosophical dualism inhibited the development of an embodied sociology in general, and health sociology in particular. The belief of the nineteenth-century 'founding fathers' that social interaction – the principle object of enquiry – could not be reduced to biology or to physiology is understood to have produced a heavy emphasis on the *social* consequences of health and illness, and to have fostered a disembodied sociology during most of the twentieth century. For example, Bryan Turner maintains that 'the legitimate rejection of biological deter-minism in favour of sociological determinism entailed . . . the exclusion of the body from the sociological imagination' (1996: 61). There is no reason to single Turner out for taking this position; it is common enough in various guises across sociology and the social sciences generally. Thus, among others, Chris Shilling (2003, 2007) claims that the body was not so much neglected in nineteenth-century sociology as an 'absent presence'. In other words, to the extent that theorists dealt with the structure and function of societies and human action, embodiment could not be ignored entirely. The argument is that the body was accorded less prominence than it deserved if a fully 'embodied sociology' was to develop. It is also widely believed that early sociologists were not interested in matters of health. In her history of the intellectual origins of medical sociology, for example, Uta Gerhardt remarks upon 'how remote in nineteenth-century sociology was the idea that a person's organic functioning was not to be taken for granted' (1989: xii). This stance will ring true for most readers. The sociology of health that we have known until very recently has not been 'embodied', nor has the wider parent discipline. But this interpretation is partial to say the least.

Given the equation of men and the social it is hardly surprising that sociology took flight from the biological body, since not to have done so would have risked its association with the natural–the emotional–illness, in other words, with woman. The flight from the body then was also a flight from supposedly female ways of being. A similar compulsion led 'the founding fathers' to neglect those women thinkers who offered an embryonic embodied sociology and fostered a collective amnesia from that point on. Harriet Martineau and Charlotte Perkins Gilman, for example, were contemporaries of Auguste Comte, Émile Durkheim, Herbert Spencer, Max Weber and others – the very sociologists for whom the body was, so it has been argued, an 'absent presence'. A consideration of their writing provides a glimpse of what could have been, had the intellectual roots of sociology been allowed to be different. This means substantially more than recovering the 'elision of the biological and social' (Fuller 2006: 81) or the corporeal in the classics (Shilling 2003; Williams and Bendelow 1998) (from which Martineau and Gilman are left out). It suggests an alternative to the conventionally disembodied origins that were embodied from the start but rendered invisible, not only by the twin problems of male dominance of the academic agenda and the philosophical dualism that sustained it, but also by a failure to recognise that this had even happened.

Early feminists of the seventeenth, eighteenth and nineteenth centuries are often portrayed as patriarchy's imitators who, by prioritising mind over matter and reason over emotion, lacked the conceptual wherewithal to mount an effective challenge to the dualistic thinking that sustained women's oppression. Certainly few commentators draw matters of health and the body into the discussion of their politics. No doubt this is why the standard starting place for accounts of feminist interest in health and the body is typically 'second wave' feminism of the 1960s and 1970s. It seems to be assumed that the endeavours of their forebears to secure political emancipation and women's access to education and the professions by arguing that women are 'just as rational as men' pretty much kept health and the body off the agenda until well into the twentieth century. Yet, even though they could not fail to be influenced by the prevailing political liberalism that deflected attention from bodily concerns, issues of health were always a forceful political undercurrent that, on occasion, rose to the surface with a vengeance in a manner that casts strong doubts over Shorter's (1982) contentions. This chapter undertakes to show that an embryonic embodied sociology and an embodied feminist politics existed as far back as the seventeenth century through women thinkers whose work collectively stretches from around the mid-seventeenth to the early twentieth century: Mary Astell, Mary Wollstonecraft, Harriet Martineau and Charlotte Perkins Gilman. Of course, these thinkers did not stand alone. Apart from the obvious reason – their attention to health – they have been chosen over others partly because of their prominence and therefore their ability to exert an influence in their own time, partly because of the accessibility of the corpus of their work to me and to readers of this book, and partly because of the breadth and depth of their work.

Reason's disciples or the body's emissaries?

Although the term 'feminist' did not come into language until the 1890s, what we now conceive as feminist thought existed well before this time and was variously known as the woman question, women's emancipation, or woman's rights (although for ease of presentation I will simply use the term feminism throughout the book). Feminism's erasure from the annals of scientific knowledge limits our ability to reconstruct women's early criticism of medicine and the 'new science' and their related attempts to understand women's circumstances and their health. However, recent feminist scholarship makes clear that criticisms of the stories the 'fathers' of the medical and social sciences wanted to tell were available even as they were being told (Keller 1997). Muted though it was, a voice of opposition was available from the start.

Feminism has a longer history than regularly is supposed. It is conventionally dated from around the mid-eighteenth century and associated with Mary Wollstonecraft. This is not the place to join the cavalcade of debate on 'who was the first feminist'. Rather, what matters is that there were women writers who, through the medium of health and illness, troubled the mind–body dualism that sustained women's oppression and made this the basis for embodied health activism. Moreover this interest was sustained – albeit in different guises and with twists and turns along the way – right through to the 1960s, the point at which 'women's health activism' and sociological interest in matters of health is usually assumed to have taken off. One of the earliest and most prominent of these women writers was Mary Astell (1666–1731).

Astell maintained that there was nothing inevitable about women's inferiority. It is 'the custom of the world', she wrote, that 'has put women, generally speaking, into a state of subjection' (Astell in Hill 1986: 72). Her treatise, *A Serious Proposal to the Ladies,* published in the 1690s (Astell 2002 [1694]), advised women to invest in much more than personal adornment. What a pity it is, she wrote, that:

> whilst your beauty casts a lustre around about, your souls which are infinitely more bright and radiant ... shou'd be suffer'd to over-run with weeds, lye fallow and neglected, unadorn'd with any grace! ... Let us learn to pride ourselves in something more excellent than the invention of a fashion' and the attraction of a man.
>
> (Astell 2002 [1694]: 54, 55)

The description of Astell as a 'dedicated Cartesian' (Smith 1982: 119) seems confirmed by such remarks as that the body 'ought to be kept in such a case as to be ready on all occasions to serve the mind' (Astell 2002 [1694]: 210). Yet she also maintained that human nature consists of the 'Union of a rational soul with a mortal body' and made it clear that it is a mistake:

> to consider either part of us singly, so as to neglect what is due the other. For if we disregard the body wholly, we pretend to live like angels whilst we are but mortals; and if we prefer or equal it to the mind we degenerate into brutes.
>
> (Ibid.: 211)

The problem, she maintained, is that 'the body very often clogs the mind in its noblest operations, especially when indulg'd' (ibid.: 210). Consequently:

> The animal spirits must be lessen'd, or rendered more calm and manageable; at least they must not be unnaturally and violently mov'd, by such a diet, or such passions, designs, and divertissements as are likely to put 'em in a ferment. Contemplation requires a governable body, a sedate and steady mind, *and the body and the mind do so reciprocally influence each other, and that we can scarce keep the one in tune if the other be out of it.*
>
> (Astell 2002 [1694]: 161, emphasis added)

The fact that governing 'natural and unavoidable' passions to which the temper of the body inclines – such as desire, fear, sorrow, hope and, above all, love – is not at all easy elevates the struggle between body and mind in Astell's work. Her 'serious proposal for the ladies' was the renunciation of sensual indulgence – including the rejection of marriage, where possible – for a chaste life of Christian stoicism. The conventional interpretation is that Astell meant women's colleges to provide the protective quarantine necessary for the cultivation of reason. However, she may also have intended them to protect women's health. Her poem *On the death of Mrs Bowes* contains the lines:

> Lost when the fatal Nuptial Knot was tie'd,
> Your Sun declin'd, when you became a Bride.
> A soul refin'd, when like your's soar'd far above
> The gross Amusements of low, Vulgar love.
>
> (Astell quoted in Perry 1979: 2)

Mrs Eleanor Bowes died aged fifteen, just three months after her marriage to a wealthy mine owner. In the opinion of Ruth Perry (1979, 1986), Astell's writing shows an awareness of the abiding association between sex and death for women and, therefore, the lurking dangers in relations with men. Every time a woman underwent the ordeal of pregnancy and childbirth in the late 1600s through to the early 1700s, she risked her life. It is very difficult to estimate maternal mortality rates for England before civil registration, which began in 1837. But drawing on the London Bills of Mortality for the lying-in hospitals (the first was established in 1739, eight years after Astell's death), Perry estimates that for every sixty safe deliveries, one woman died. If a woman delivered six children (which was not uncommon among the wealthy), she had at least a 10 per cent chance of dying, probably higher. And there was not only death to be feared but also in the wake of birth there was the prospect of life-long pain and chronic illness from infection or from a ruptured or prolapsed uterus. Puerperal fever, a newly recognised disease of unknown aetiology, was a particular cause for alarm. Reporting on a mid-eighteenth-century outbreak in the Jordanne Valley of France, one doctor found it made women so fearful that 'young girls recoiled from marriage' (cited in Gélis 1991: 246). The seclusion of life with other women therefore 'had the real utility of sparing life and health' (Perry 1979: 36). In sum, the twin problem of the conventional association between men and reason and male power over women's bodies meant that Astell had to work hard to establish women's right to reason by actively engaging with bodily concerns even at the same time that she shunned what she saw as the burdens of the flesh. This brought women's bodily health into – rather than excluded it from – her vision.

Astell was staunchly conservative and opposed to class levelling, her advocacy of education for women extending only to people like herself (Perry 1986). Born almost thirty years after Astell's death, Mary Wollstonecraft (1759–97), combined the 'woman of reason' with a decidedly radical politics. Her *Vindication of the Rights of Woman* (1992 [1792]) was published more than a hundred years on from Astell's *Serious Proposal* and in a markedly different social and economic climate. By the late eighteenth century, the Enlightenment had bequeathed a new attitude to educated Europeans, a new questioning of authority, the application of reason through the new science and a seemingly unwavering belief in social progress and improvement. At first glance, the appeal of the following changes for women seems self-evident:

> They experienced an expansive sense of power over nature and themselves: the pitiless cycles of epidemics, famines, risky life and early death, devastating war and uneasy peace – the treadmill of human existence – seemed to be yielding at last to the application of critical intelligence. Fear of change, up to that time nearly universal, was giving way to fear of stagnation; the word innovation, traditionally an effective term of abuse, became a word of praise . . . There seemed to be little doubt that in the struggle of man against nature, the balance of power was strongly in favour of man.
>
> (Gray quoted in Hamilton 1992: 40)

Yet, as this quotation inadvertently signals, the balance of power truly was in favour of man (not woman), for even though the Enlightenment raised the possibility of a brave new world for women, by the turn of the nineteenth century it was widely maintained that biological difference made human rights sex-specific and inapplicable to women. Wollstonecraft's work was a powerful attack on this conviction. Although she shared the political views of radical male thinkers of her time, she vehemently opposed their treatment of women. Jean-Jacques Rousseau in particular was subject to strident criticism. How could he argue that inequalities are socially created and in the same breath, so to speak, also claim that the inequalities between men and women – and male superiority – are natural? Wollstonecraft specifically challenged Rousseau's views on moral education expounded in the book *Émile* (1966 [1762]), which advanced the belief that women should not be educated, except in virtue and in the care of men. If women's condition is natural, then why, she asked, do they have to be trained into this 'non productive vacuousness'?

Since the body posed an immanent risk to reason there is an inevitable tension in the mind–body relationship in Astell's work. For Wollstonecraft the body is far more flexible, poised to be fit for the (rational) mind, but hindered by social convention. The bodily strength that supposedly gives man a natural superiority over woman is to all intents and purposes irrelevant. It is how we respond socially to these differences that really matters. Thus, she asks, why does it follow that it is natural for woman 'to labour to become still weaker than nature intended her to be?' Why are women 'so infatuated as to be proud of a defect?' (Wollstonecraft 1992 [1792]: 125, 127). Her answer lies in the social conventions that induce women to 'feign a sickly delicacy' in order to ensure their husbands' affections (ibid.: 112). Wollstonecraft was particularly concerned to rehabilitate those bourgeois women whose once productive role in the domestic economy had been replaced by economic dependence with the rise of capitalism (Eisenstein 1981). Since she believed that 'dependence of body naturally produced dependence of mind', there was little hope for women who, quite literally and so unnecessarily, were not only made slaves to their bodies but gloried in their subjection (Wollstonecraft 1992: 130). She was adamant that 'sedentary employments render the majority of women sickly – and false notions of female excellence make them proud of this delicacy, though it be another fetter, that by calling attention continually to the body, cramps the activity of the mind' (ibid.: 171). Thus:

> confined . . . in cages like the feathered race, they have nothing to do but to plume themselves, and stalk with mock majesty from perch to perch. It is true that they are provided with food and raiment, for which they neither toil nor spin; but health, liberty, and virtue are given in exchange.
>
> (Wollstonecraft 1992 [1792]: 146)

She exhorted those responsible for the education of girls not to destroy their constitutions with mistaken ideals of female beauty and manners. We should hear nothing of women's fragility, she wrote, 'if girls were allowed to take sufficient exercise, and not confined in close rooms till their muscles are relaxed and their digestion destroyed' (ibid.: 154). The ability to educate women for independence is therefore intimately connected with their bodily well-being for Wollstonecraft.

The tag 'reason's disciples' in the heading to this section of the chapter is borrowed from the title of Hilda Smith's (1982) book on seventeenth-century feminists (though I believe the spirit of the expression carries through to the eighteenth century and beyond). Its use is intended to convey that the right to reason was of utmost concern for these women. As noted earlier, since they were bound to pursue women's right to education and to employment outside the home, the conception of 'reason's disciples' seems appropriate. But it does not thereby follow that they were patriarchy's imitators, drawn away from 'things bodily' and wrong-footed by opting into, rather than challenging, the dualisms that would continue to oppress them. Although it was not always in the foreground, they were concerned to show that women's physical and mental ill health was socially formed and not biologically given. It is in this sense that I have counterposed 'reason's disciples' with the less eloquent notion of the 'body's emissaries'. Yet to ask, as I have done, whether 'first wave' feminists were 'reason's disciples' *or* the 'body's emissaries' also misses the point. Showing that states of health and illness arose from the social relations within society placed mind and body in contiguity. This budding sense of embodied health (involving a fusing of mind and body) held out the potential of a health activism that, if it could not yet undermine, would at least trouble the association of women with the negative and devalued (the natural–body–emotion–illness).

Health fiction

Getting their writing into print and daring to do so under their own name was a sizeable challenge for women. Fiction was a far more acceptable genre than the political tract, where few would have dared to venture, even if it was possible, given the propensity to trounce women's ideas through ridicule of their persona (Wollstonecraft, for example, suffered dearly in this respect). Writing for periodicals, magazines and annuals was one of the few respectable ways for educated women to make a living and a vital source of income for the single or widowed (Jump 1998).

Fiction traditionally has been located in a different part of the academy to the social sciences. Yet the writings of women such as Jane Austen, Elizabeth Gaskell, Charlotte Brontë and George Eliot (the pen name of Marian Evans) give a sense of gender relations largely absent from social sciences' 'founding fathers' (Deegan 1997; Evans 2003). There is some debate over whether these, and other women writers of the time, can be seen as feminists. Some are of the opinion that the politics of the pen mean that 'woman author' and 'feminist author' are synonymous. For example, Jane Austen, who customarily has been seen as apolitical and uninterested in the politics of her day, has recently been endowed with feminist intent. Equally, it has been argued that it takes too much reinterpretation to make her fit the feminist mould (see discussion in Brooke 1999; Kirkham 1983; Looser 1995). But, following Devony Looser, I believe the important point is that the novels of Austen and others provide 'significant commentary on what it means to perform the subject position "woman"' (1995: 9). What really matters is not so much whether an author 'is' or 'is not' a feminist but the working of gender and health politics in her novels.

There is growing interest in the commentary of women novelists on health and illness (see, for example, Bailin 1994; Frawley 2004; Wiltshire 1997; Wood 2001). With the poetic licence that the novel afforded, they were fully able to explore illness as a social pathology, that is, as arising from the context of their characters' lives. Many read widely on medical and related science matters, both to give credence to their work and to mount a plausible challenge to medical understandings. For instance, George Eliot diligently researched aspects of bodily illness in preparation for *Middlemarch* (Chase 1984; Wood 2001) and is credited as probably the first novelist to portray the new kind of doctor that was emerging at the time 'with historical precision' (Harvey 1985: 19). At first glance, titles such as Jane Austen's *Pride and Prejudice* and *Sense and Sensibility* (published in 1813 and 1811 respectively) connote a preoccupation with matters of the mind rather than the body. But as John Wiltshire argues, it is not possible to conceive of the relationship between her characters and their worlds 'as simply between mind or consciousness and external reality' (1997: 9). Illness is a vehicle for the social tensions of society, which are played out in the symptoms of characters who literally embody their society and often suffer the consequences.

It has been remarked that there is 'scarcely a Victorian fictional narrative without its ailing protagonist, its depiction of a sojourn in the sickroom' (Bailin 1994: 5). Bearing in mind that episodes of interest in women's health frequently coincide with periods of significant change in their social and economic roles (Weisman 1998), it is instructive that characters often enter the sickroom because they have experienced a personal crisis and become separated from the social roles and norms that have defined their lives. As Carroll Smith-Rosenberg (1985: 208) discusses for female hysteria, this illness 'became one way in which conventional women could express – in most cases unconsciously – dissatisfaction with one or more aspects of their lives', most notably the confines of the wife–mother role. In the manner of the later concept of the 'sick role' by sociologist Talcott Parsons (1950), the sickroom is a sanctioned form of protection from the 'discontinuities of experience and frustrations of communal life' (Bailin

1994: 18). Given that women's domain of the home was traversed by others with impunity, the sickroom could provide them, quite literally, with the only 'room of their own'. For example, in *Ruth* (1985 [1853]), Elizabeth Gaskell describes the invalid's room as having an atmosphere of peace and encouragement that affected all who entered it. Since women were pressed both into sickness and into ministering to the sick, the sickroom might seem an unlikely place of self-empowerment. But, despite the suffering therein, sickroom sequestration was particularly important for women as a 'kind of forcing ground of the self – a conventional rite of passage issuing in personal, moral, or social recuperation' (Bailin 1994: 5).[1]

While Austen, Gaskell and others were debatably 'feminist' in intent, there was an important minority who engaged in *both* fiction *and* political writing in the name of women. For example, George Eliot translated Ludwig Feuerbach's *The Essence of Christianity* (the only work to appear under her birth name) and reflected on Wollstonecraft's *Vindication* (Eliot 1855). But there is perhaps no body of scholarly, fictional and autobiographical writing more conducive to the union of sociological thought with critical reflection on health and on women's position than that of Harriet Martineau and Charlotte Perkins Gilman.

Martineau: the sickroom and gender politics

Harriet Martineau (1802–76) is known principally within sociology for her English translation of Auguste Comte's six-volume work, *Cours de Philosophie Positive* (Comte 1830–42; Martineau 1853).[2] Reflecting on this task, she remarked that she 'should never enjoy any thing so much again' (Martineau 1877: 390). Comte was so pleased, he had the work back-translated into French. Important though this and other accolades were, it is testimony to the erasure of women from the history of sociology that Martineau is far better known today for this translation than for her own sociological works (Madoo Lengermann and Niebrugge-Brantley 1998, 2003). Her acclaimed *Society in America* (1962 [1836/1837]) and *How to Observe Morals and Manners* (1838) appeared well before Comte's *Cours*.

Martineau identified health and the position of women as two of the most important sociologically observable patterns of relationships between people (or what she called 'manners') that reveal a society's 'morals' (or what we would now call its norms and values). Thus health status was an indicator that could be used to interpret the wider character of a society:

> one character of morals and manners prevails where the greater number die young, and another where they die old; one where they are cut off by hardship; another where they waste away under a lingering disease; and yet another where they abide their full time, and then come to their graves like a shock of corn in its season.
>
> (Martineau 1838: 166)

Her feminism is revealed in the anomalies between a society's declared and its actual morals. She believed that 'the degree of degradation of woman is as good a test as the moralist can adopt for ascertaining the state of domestic morals in any country' (ibid.: 174). The conditions of both women and slaves – Martineau was an outspoken abolitionist – were documented in *Society in America*, which was the result of two years of extensive travel away from her English homeland to converse with and observe women and men from a range of social backgrounds across the United States.[3] She found that American society was operating under the fallacy of distinct masculine and feminine qualities of hardy men and gentle women. How, she asks, 'is the restricted and dependent state of women to be reconciled with the proclamation that "all are endowed by their Creator with certain unalienable rights; that among these are life, liberty and the pursuit of happiness"?'(Martineau 1962: 308).[4]

A blending of narrative fiction and realism made Martineau's ideas far more accessible than would ever have been possible through a narrowly academic style (Logan 2002; Sanders 1986). If, as she put it, 'good and bad health is both cause and effect of good and bad morals' (Martineau 1838: 163), then neither health status nor the status of women are natural givens. For example, she maintained that the reason why the health of nineteenth-century schoolgirls was generally worse than that of schoolboys had relatively little to do with their biology and everything to do with 'the unequal development of the faculties' (Martineau 1861: 22). Thus:

> there is too much intellectual acquisition, though not too much mental exercise . . . and there is an almost total absence of physical education. If the muscles were called upon as strenuously as the memory to show what they could do, the long train of school-girls who institute the romance of the coming generation would flock merrily into ten thousand homes, instead of parting off – some to gladden their homes, certainly, but too many to the languid lot of invalidism, or to the actual sick-room; while an interminable procession of them is for ever on its way to the cemetery – the foremost dropping into the grave while the number is kept up from behind.
>
> (Martineau 1861: 22–3)

As we have seen, Wollstonecraft (1992 [1792]) similarly reflected writing towards the end of the eighteenth century. However, Martineau paid far more attention to health than her feminist predecessors. The health of women of working age was a particular concern (see Logan 2002). By focusing on specific occupations and 'stations in life', she drew attention to the causes of needless mortality and 'the prevalent imperfections of health, for which society is answerable' in a series of articles in the periodical *Once a Week* (Martineau 1861: 267). For example, she was concerned that the needlewoman's conditions of work made her vulnerable to spinal disease and blindness. She believed that turning over all of one's time to child care is far from natural or good for women. The indefatigable devotion of live-in governesses to the education and care of their charges is 'cause enough for a perpetual fever of mind and wear of nerves, leading to illness, to failure of temper, to a resort to stimulants by slow degrees'. In other words, it is enough to drive a governess to drink. Insult is quite literally added to injury since 'the salary does not afford any prospect of a sufficient provision when health and energy is worn out' (ibid.: 195, 196).

Martineau 'viewed fiction as an experimental mode in which the theoretical principles of the social sciences can be worked out' (Hill and Hoecker-Drysdale 2003: 19). In Martineau's novel *Deerbrook* (2004 [1839]) the sickness of society, manifest in the petty rivalries and jealousies of English village life, is disclosed in contests over medical knowledge and the trials and tribulations of the village doctor Edward Hope and his family. At the heart of the novel is the harnessing of women's chances in life to their marriage prospects. Health is integral to this plot. Doctor Hope fails to appreciate the domestic 'dis-ease' to which his new young wife Hester falls prey. As she explains to her sister: 'life is a blank to me. I have no hope left. I am neither wiser, nor better, nor happier, for God having given me all that should make a woman what I meant to be' (ibid.: 242). Hester is only rescued from her growing malaise when called to action in the care of the sick – and becomes a true companion to her husband – when the fever comes to the village (England had experienced a real-life cholera epidemic in the early 1830s). Governess Maria Young, however, loses the prospect of marriage altogether after being disabled and subject to a life of pain following an accident. This almost certainly reflects an episode from Martineau's childhood when she was seven years old, when a friend of her own age lost a leg in an accident. She reflects that this event 'influenced my whole mind and character more than almost all other influences together' (letter in Sanders 1990: 60). In *Deerbrook*, Philip Enderby, who had a close affection for Maria before her accident, rather shamefully admits that he recalls rejoicing after her accident that his 'esteem for her had not passed into a warmer feeling', that is, to love (Martineau 2004 [1839]: 332). Unbeknownst to Enderby, Maria is still in love with him. Even though Maria is able to make her way in life as a governess, she fears terribly for her old age as the threat of worsening health endangers her livelihood.

In both her fictional and sociological writing Martineau threw the equation of illness–natural–women into relief by demonstrating the social basis of their ill health. This did not involve a flight from biology, but rather an appreciation of the embodied nature of experience, that is, what is social is simultaneously corporeal. This does not mean to say that her thinking was free of tensions. Mind/body dualism was under wider challenge at the time (Winter 1998) and perceptions of the nature of males and females in flux. As Mary Poovey discusses, the gender ideologies of any period are always 'in the making' and, therefore, 'open to revision, dispute, and the emergence of oppositional formulations' (1988: 3). This found expression in Martineau's writing on chronic illness.

Life in the sickroom

Martineau's writing on the experience of illness had very personal origins. She lost most of her hearing at the age of twelve and used an ear trumpet as an adult.[5] Aged 37 in 1839, she became unwell with a gynaecological complaint while travelling in Venice. The consensus is that she was suffering from a prolapsed uterus caused by a benign ovarian cyst, although this was not clear at the time. Between 1840 and 1844 she lived the life of an invalid. Secluded in her sickroom in the coastal town of Tynemouth in the north of England, she wrote her personal account, *Life in the Sickroom* (2003 [1844]). As Ann Oakley has recently written, within the academy autobiographical writing 'is often seen negatively, as a form of inexcusable self-indulgence' (2007: 23). Yet 'writing is a way to assert the authenticity of the self . . . Through the text, we reclaim the body; we have some hope of owning and integrating the experience of damage' (ibid.: 152–3).

Life in the Sickroom needs to be read in the context of two nineteenth-century enthusiasms: first, for the use of the sickroom metaphor in fiction, mentioned earlier; and second, for advice-giving. It self-consciously appeals to the fraternity of experience and evinces a strong desire to instruct others (Frawley 2004: 247). Thus Martineau wrote in a letter of 1834 concerning her 'letter to the deaf': 'people with all infirmities are reading my sermon. As a lady said to me, "we all have our deafness"' (Martineau in Sanders 1990: 43–4). Although *Life in the Sickroom* has much in common with the popular genre of health advice literature of the time, it stands out for its wider sociological interpretation of the invalid condition (Annandale 2007; Frawley 2004). In the literal sense of seeing, Martineau writes with wonder of the potential to fill a volume with the simple detail of life witnessed from her one back-room window, often with the aid of her telescope, such as the comings and goings of her neighbours and the town's sailors. Being set apart from the 'disturbing bustles of life in the world' provides the invalid with the singular opportunity to contemplate many sides of a question, the ability not only to see much farther than one used to, but also much farther than 'others do on subjects of interest, which involve general principles' (Martineau 2003 [1844]: 117). Sociological insight is forged through the conviction that, since invalids are denied slices of actual life, they think through a blending of 'history, life and speculation', which, in a previously healthy life, would have constituted decidedly separate 'departments of study'. In her own words: 'history becomes like actual life; life becomes comprehensive as history, and abstract as speculation' (ibid.: 91).

The syncretic sociological insight that emerges from the invalid experience is accentuated in Martineau's view by the alertness to the mind/body relationship that accompanies illness, especially its companion, pain. She anticipates present-day discourse on the taken-for-granted, or absent presence of the fit and healthy body, remarking, for example, in a discussion of the maid-of-all-work that:

> she does not think about her bodily condition at all; for there are no aches and pains to remind her. Some people go through life without ever having felt their lungs; and others are unaware, except by rational evidence, that they have a stomach.
>
> (Martineau 1861: 160)

As Simon Williams and Gillian Bendelow explain:

> while at an *analytical* level the study of illness, pain and suffering demand dissolution of former dualistic modes of thinking, in drawing attention to the relatedness of self and world, mind and body, inside and out, we must also account for the enduring power and qualities of these dichotomies at the *experiential* level of suffering.
>
> (1998: 136, emphasis in the original)

Martineau was acutely aware of this. She wrote that bodily pain can so affect the mind that it loses all its gaiety and, by disuse, almost forgets its sense of enjoyment. But pain can also act as a relief from the gnawing misery of the invalid's mind; thus, 'the more restless is the distressed body, the more at ease does the spirit appear' (Martineau 1844: 113). Aware of the counterintuitive nature of her claim, she explains that the sick person is never as happy as when they feel their paroxysms of pain coming on, for they know that the aftermath will bring relative ease. In this sense, the body appeases the distress of the mind. Appeasement also works in the other direction as the power of ideas offers respite from bodily pain. For Martineau, the sick vindicated 'the supremacy of mind over body' (ibid.: 129). This signalled the power of being over doing (Frawley 1997, 2004), the crucial recognition that despite their liabilities, the sick can still *be* even though they cannot *do*. *Life in the Sickroom* therefore was an attempt to overturn the idea that the sickroom was for those who had opted out of life and to instate it instead as a platform for direct political intervention in the world.

Martineau attributed her eventual return to health to mesmerism, which was at the height of its popular interest at the time. Her celebrity ensured her cure was a nationwide sensation (Cooter 1991) and a very public challenge to doctors whose new medical techniques were premised on a quite different understanding of the body (Winter 1998). To Martineau's distress, her brother-in-law, Dr Thomas Greenhow, who had treated her up to this point, published her case without her permission in a shilling pamphlet in 1845. Along with others, he maintained that as the ovarian cyst that had caused her uterus to prolapse had grown, it had forced her uterus back up into her pelvis, and this coincided with the mesmeric treatment (Annandale 2007; Ryall 2000). Martineau fiercely contested this, remarking 'I was never lower than immediately before I made trial of mesmerism' (Martineau 1844: 4).

Although, on the surface, mesmerism appears to vindicate the power of mind over body and thereby substantiate mind/body dualism, a closer inspection discloses a more complex relationship. For Martineau, mesmerism was the key to a social scientific understanding of the mind/body relationship. First of all, it was not simply a matter of mind *over* body but the power of mind *and* body (Martineau 1844). Mesmeric practice varied from practitioner to practitioner, but its basic principle was the power of one person to affect another's mind and body. It displayed the spectacle of 'human beings intimately connected to each other by invisible substances', of their identities extending beyond the visible border of the body and flowing into one another (Winter 1998: 117). It was conceived as a force of nature that could restore equilibrium to body and mind. As Alison Winter puts it:

> through the direct action of a force of nature on her nervous system, Martineau had attained access to the 'very laws of life' and the source of all beliefs about the world, and was able to understand how they related to one another.
>
> (1998: 223)

This accorded with her wider sociological endeavour, which involved a naturalistic approach to explanation, 'integrating factors of the biophysical environment with the social and economic' (McDonald 2003: 156). This brings us back to Martineau's sympathy with Comtean positivism. Although she took issue with Comte's views on women, his racism and his vision of a hierarchically organised society, she shared his conception of the interconnections of the individual, the social and the natural world and the search for natural laws of human existence. Sociology could uncover these connections by empirical observation and this was facilitated by the development of the human mind away from theological and metaphysical forms of knowledge towards positivistic understanding (Hoecker-Drysdale 2003).[6]

Martineau's writing on the invalid condition therefore encompasses the themes of her wider work. It demonstrates her search for a syncretic and empirical understanding of the social world and the place of the individual within it. The connection between the circumstances of women's lives, particularly their working lives, and their health status is very clear. Her articles in *Once a Week* were direct attempts to improve matters. Her supposition that the individual experience of illness is a platform for political intervention is apparent in her advocacy of mesmerism, which was a challenge to the establishing medical orthodoxy. As Caroline Roberts (2002) points out, somnambulists such as Martineau's maid, Jane, were mostly women and, moreover, women who were physically and emotionally weakened. Ostensibly bound by animal sensibilities or their biology, mesmerism appeared to be demonstrating that women had more self-command than generally was supposed.

Yet, arguably Martineau's most important work in this regard, *Life in the Sickroom*, is not overtly feminist insofar as it appears to be directed equally to men and to women and does not openly confront the medical treatment of women. It could be said that this apparent neutrality made it possible for her to undercut the conventional association between invalidism, passivity, powerlessness and women by emphasising the unique agency that the sick role cultivates for all. An equally plausible reading is that Martineau's outwardly separate discourse on illness and discourse on gender in *Life in the Sickroom* is that they were bound to act in concert. As the disparagement of her persona by medical men testifies, her very public profile meant that neither her personal nor her sociological accounts of illness could fail to resonate but in gendered terms. Health politics were always to some extent gender politics simply because 'illness' and 'woman' were always to some extent stitched together. Obviously this was not unassailable since the connection could always be challenged and unpicked. But the threat of repair was always there, and this meant that illness could never actually be gender-neutral. The argument that follows from this reading is that since women and illness were part of the same dense cultural fabric, they had to be overturned together. Therefore, by turning the conventional association of illness with inactivity into mental activity – what is more, activity with privileged insight – Martineau simultaneously also converted the companionate – women – into active beings with privileged insight.

Gilman: living and dying in a 'man-made world'

Born when Martineau was in her late fifties and a continent away in the United States, Charlotte Perkins Gilman (1860–1935) was far less reticent in pointing directly to the damage that 'the patriarchate' wrought on the female body and laying some of the blame at the door of the male medical profession. Much like Martineau before her, she 'swept through her era in a blaze of notoriety' (Deegan 1997: 8). From academic works to journalism, novels and short stories, Gilman brought a blend of sociological and feminist insight to the problem of women's health. The heart of her concern was what she called the 'excessive sex distinction' within late nineteenth-century American society. Men had created a masculine culture in excess, premised on a seemingly natural division by sex (biology), which had surged over all its natural boundaries and emblazoned itself 'across every act of life, so that every step of the human creature is marked "male" or "female"' (Gilman 1966 [1898]: 52–3). In developing this position, Gilman drew appreciatively upon the work of sociologist Lester Ward, who at the time was arguing that 'male and female differences which the androcentric view suggests are innate [. . .] are the result of the long subjection of women that has exaggerated their differences from men' (Palmeri 1983: 103).[7] Gilman explained that:

> when we say *men, man, manly, manhood* and all the other masculine derivatives, we have in the background of our minds a huge vague crowded picture of the world and its activities . . . And when we say *women*, we think *female* – the sex.
> (Gilman 1998 [1915]: 116, 117, emphasis original)

In other words, this reduced women to their biology while allowing men to be so much more. The result is women's economic dependence on men, from which flows all manner of assaults on their well-being. As Gilman put it in the serialised article, 'Our Androcentric culture', 'we have so far lived and suffered and died in a man-made world'.[8]

The institution of marriage reflects women's dependence and, more often than not, is the root of their physical and mental deterioration. The marriage ceremony commonly appears in Gilman's writing as 'the precise moment that the woman passes from a vigorous, healthy girlhood into a married state which will bring physical decline' (Beer 1998: 63; see also Beer 1997). This conviction undoubtedly grew out of her own sorry experience. She was a vigorous and healthy young woman herself – she enjoyed nothing more than going to the gymnasium, and even ran the '7 minute mile' (Hill 1980) – but her health began to decline soon after her marriage in 1884 at the age of twenty-four, and fell to greater depths with the pregnancy that soon followed. When her daughter was five months old, she wrote in her diary thus: 'every morning the same hopeless waking . . . the same weary drag. To die mere cowardice. Retreat impossible, escape impossible' (Gilman quoted in Hill 1980: 128). She admonished herself, remarking, 'you had health and strength and hope and glorious work before you – and you threw it away' (Gilman 1963 [1935]: 91). In 1887, and with 'the utmost confidence', Gilman sought help from the eminent Philadelphian neurologist, Silas Weir Mitchell and underwent his six-week 'rest cure' (ibid.: 95). She had written to him in advance with a summary of her case, an action that, ominously, he dismissed as self-conceit. Weir Mitchell advised her, as he did other women, to devote her life to domestic work and her child and to confine herself to no more than two hours of intellectual work each day. He particularly warned her to 'never touch pen, brush or pencil as long as you live' (ibid.: 96). Trying for over three months to obey these instructions led Gilman near the borderline of utter mental ruin. Her torment was such that she would 'crawl into remote closets and under beds – to hide from the grinding pressure of that profound distress' (Gilman quoted in Hill 1980: 149). She later explained that 'using the remnants of intelligence that remained, and helped by a wise friend, I cast the noted specialist's advice to the winds and went to work again' (Gilman 1913a: 86).

Her experience of 'nervous breakdown' was later told in the chilling autobiographical novella, *The Yellow Wallpaper* (Gilman 1973 [1892]). The narrator has been taken by her doctor husband and sister-in-law to a rather broken down mansion for a rest to aid her recovery from nervous illness. She describes being secluded under the 'careful and loving' direction of her husband in a room in this rented house covered in horrible, malodorous yellow wallpaper. Mirroring Gilman's own experience, this young wife and mother wishes more than anything to work, but the medical advice is that she does nothing. Within the wallpaper's sprawling and flamboyant patterns she sees the form of a woman trapped and trying to break free. The woman struggles, but as much as she tries to break through, the pattern in the wallpaper strangles her, turns her upside down and makes her eyes white. On her last day in the house, the narrator undertakes to help her. While Gilman was able, quite literally, to write herself out of madness, the narrator is not so fortunate: she begins to 'read' the wallpaper and eventually descends into madness, coming to believe that she is herself the woman who has escaped from inside it.

Gilman recognised her own recovery to be an exception. She defended the tale, which some believed was itself enough to send people insane, by explaining that it was written to 'save people being driven crazy' and, what is more, that 'it worked' (Gilman 1913a: 86). This was part of her wider ambition to use 'health fiction' to inform about health problems and cultivate women's agency (Cutter 2001). A specific desire was to reach Weir Mitchell 'and convince him of the error of his ways' (Gilman 1913b: 88). Gilman sent him a copy, but received no reply. She recounts that 'many years later, I met someone who knew close friends of Dr Mitchell's who said he had told them that he changed his treatment of nervous prostration since reading "*The Yellow Wallpaper*"' (Gilman 1913b: 88–9). However, this may have been wishful thinking since Julie Bates Dock (1998) reports that she could find no evidence of this and that, indeed, he still propounded his thesis and methods years later.

For Gilman, good health resulted from an 'equipoise of soul and body' (1916a: 68) that rested on a felt harmony between the individual and their social environment. She believed that for this to happen, individuals need to be 'convinced that the work they are doing is necessary and right'. If they are not convinced, 'the effect on their nervous system is disastrous' (ibid.: 69). She believed that finding this balance was difficult enough for people generally given the social changes taking place in society of the time, such as urbanisation, the expansion of the cities, and an increasing pace of life. But for women, it was magnified many times over. The new opportunities in the world of work were out there, but hardly within their grasp as they were hindered 'by the cold and cruel opposition of the other sex' (ibid.: 74). Under these circumstances, she believed that people should not have been asking, as was the tendency at the time, why so *many* women experience nervous breakdown, but why so *few*.

In the utopian novel *Herland* (1998 [1915]), Gilman envisaged an alternative world that sustains women's health. The three American men who 'discover' the land had expected to find hysteria but realised instead 'a standard of health and vigour, a calmness of temper' (ibid.: 69). Freed from the real world opposition of male and female and living in a woman-only environment, sickness was almost wholly unknown, 'so much so that a previously high development in what we call the "science of medicine" had become practically a lost art. They were a clean-bred, vigorous lot, having the best of care, the most perfect living condition always' (ibid.: 61). Parthenogenetic, the women had borne only female children for two thousand years. In *Herland*, the visitors fall in love and Van marries Ellador. The sequel, *With Her in Ourland* (Gilman 1916b), follows the travels of Ellador and Van as they leave 'herland' for the real world, or 'ourland'. As they reach Europe, the First World War is raging. Ellador grows paler and harder by the day as she endeavours to understand the hitherto unimaginable. The war is sickening her body as she absorbs the pain of others. She trains as a physician, meets and talks with economists, psychologists and sociologists, and uses her sensibilities to diagnose the world's ills.

In these utopian novels Gilman sets up an opposition of her own, between male individualism in the real, or 'ourworld', and female communitarianism in 'herland'. Yes, these are women with a difference, economically powerful and able to work in male-defined domains. But they are also essentially nurturing, both of their young and of each other. Men, by contrast, are portrayed as individualistic and resistant to change (Beer 1997). There is, then, a sense of female superiority grounded in a biologically based 'maternal instinct' (Deegan 1997). But by contrasting Ellador and Van's experience in 'herland' and in 'ourland' Gilman may have intended to press the point that women are not fixed by their natures; rather, their natures are responsive to the social organisation of society. Moreover, it is possible for men to change, as witnessed in the enlightenment of the character of Van (who, notably, is a sociologist).[9] In *With Her in Ourland* and elsewhere, such as the serialised work, 'Our Androcentric culture', Gilman advances a liberal humanist position, calling for 'a change from the dominance of one sex to the equal power of two'.[10] It was highly unnatural, as she put it, to break society into two. She believed that, 'in the economic world, excessive masculinity, in its fierce competition and primitive individualism; and excessive femininity, in its inordinate consumption and hindering conservatism; have reached a stage where they work more evil than good' (Gilman 1966 [1898]: 139–40). The dichotomy between male and female, masculine and feminine, and producer and consumer had grown so out of all proportion that it contained the seeds of its own destruction. Quite simply, sex distinction and the economic dependence of women on men that accompanies it threatens the survival of the species (Palmeri 1983).

As noted earlier, like Astell and Martineau and others before her, Gilman persistently marked out marriage as a turning point in women's health. In the short story 'The vintage', Leslie, a young woman of 'blazing health', surrenders her own health and that of her children (who are born dead or deformed) when she marries Rodger Moore, a man with syphilis, and dies totally unaware of what has ailed her (Gilman 1916c). Moore's doctor – a previous suitor of Leslie – urges him to reconsider the marriage, but he will hear nothing of it. But what can the doctor do? 'He was a physician with a high sense of professional honour. The physician must not betray his patient . . .' (ibid.: 299). So he held his tongue. Through this short story Gilman exposed this 'vintage tradition' as a pretence. Privacy was invaded regularly with other infectious diseases, such as smallpox and scarlet fever; and 'if you tell the doctor that you have leprosy – there's nothing sacred about that. Off with you to the pest house, at any cost of pain and shame to you or your family'.[11] Therefore it is not really confidentiality that is at work here, but men's protection of each other, their apparent lack of regard for women's health and their bid to silence them by excluding them from knowledge and, consequently, personal agency (Cutter 2001).[12]

In England at this time, Christabel Pankhurst (1880–1958) was also arguing that marriage was a 'matter of appalling danger to women' given that the large majority were wholly ignorant of the risks posed to them by male promiscuity (1913: 63). She reported that women struck down by illness within days or weeks of their wedding had their sex organs removed under the cover of a lie that they were suffering from appendicitis. She said she had it on medical authority that 'out of 1,000 abdominal operations on women, 950 – all save 50! – were the result of conditions due to gonorrhoea' (ibid.: 43). Women were not natural invalids as they had been led to believe; they were invalids because they were victims of sexual disease. Indeed, she contended that it was largely due to the ravages of gonorrhoea that 'womanhood has itself come to be looked upon as a disease' (ibid.: 84). Making a firm statement of embodied health politics, Pankhurst remarked:

> what a cruel mockery it is that men have alleged the very weakness of which their behaviour is a cause as a reason why women should be condemned to political inferiority!
>
> (Pankhurst 1913: 95)

For Pankhurst the cure was two-fold: 'Votes for Women, which will give to women more self-reliance and a stronger economic position, and chastity for men' (ibid.: 37).[13] Between 1864 and the repeal of the English Contagious Diseases Acts in 1886, 'medical policemen' had the right to identify, examine, detain for up to three months and compulsorily treat women who were suspected of spreading disease through prostitution. For men who consorted with prostitutes, there was no such punishment. The Royal Commission on the Administration of the Acts of 1871 justified the differential treatment of women on the grounds that 'with one sex [women] the offence is committed as a matter of gain; with the other [men] it is an irregular indulgence of natural impulse' (quoted in Spender 1982: 472; for a wider discussion see Walkowitz 1980). Martineau, who was then in her mid-sixties, came out of retirement to petition for women's civil liberty and the repeal of the Acts. Elizabeth Blackwell (the first woman to obtain a medical degree) professed that her involvement moulded the whole of her future life, so much so that her eyes were 'suddenly opened, never to be closed again' to the 'social degradation produced by the double standard of morality' and the 'direful purchase of women which is really the greatest obstacle to the progress of the race' (Blackwell 1977 [1895]: 242–3). In common with many other *fin-de-siècle* feminists, Gilman was ambivalent about birth control. On the one hand, she was aware that unchecked pregnancy and caring for a large number of children was a danger to women's health. On the other, it seemed to provide men with sexual licence. Nonetheless she advocated women's choice and spoke before the US Congress hearings for legalised birth control. More generally, she was worried by the growth of women's sexual freedom and felt that there was no reason for them to rival the promiscuity of men in their lives (Gilman 1923: 1963).

'New women'

While the concerns raised by Gilman and her contemporaries about women's sexual relations with men, venereal disease and the dangers of marriage struck a chord with many, Gilman lamented that where young women were concerned, this was falling on deaf ears. Writing in 1923, aged seventy-three, she professed 'small patience' with the 'new women', whom she described in a letter to her daughter as 'painted, powdered, high-heeled, cigarette-smoking idiots'. Of course, the specific link between smoking and ill health was not known at this time. But on the new popularity of smoking, she exclaimed: 'to deliberately take up an extra vice – or bad habit – just to show off – imbecile' (Gilman, cited in Lane 1997: 342). Although she would not have intended her comments to be taken in quite this way, Gilman provides a glimpse of what was to become a recurring theme over the years, namely that when given their freedom, women often lapse into 'bad habits' (see Chapter 6). A letter writer to the *Daily Mail* newspaper in 1906, for example, claimed that women who smoke 'are slack and casual about everything. They neglect their homes and families; they neglect their social duties; their God they have ceased to pay any heed to; their husband's authority they reject with ridicule' (quoted in Hilton 2000: 141). The First World War was a watershed both in the emancipation of women and the spread of smoking among them. Attitudes started to change and women began to use the cigarette as a weapon of challenge to traditional ideas about their behaviour (Amos and Haglund 2000). In 1921, the Great American Tobacco company hired several young women 'to smoke their "torches of freedom" (*Lucky Strikes*) as they marched down Fifth Avenue protesting against women's inequality' (ibid.: 5).

Gilman's critical reflections on the 'new woman' of the 1920s and 1930s are prophetic in many ways. She pointed with pride to their growing economic freedom, which she associated not only with their increased life expectancy but also with a new kind of 'life cycle', remarking that 'today they have longer childhood, longer youth, and maturity holds on steadily, with health and strength, ambition and enjoyment, well into what used to be mere fireside knitting time' (Gilman 1923: 734). But she also remarked that she had expected 'better things of women than they have shown' (Gilman 1963 [1935]: 318). She believed that social change had brought losses, pointing in particular to 'certain very conspicuous and decidedly evil features in the behaviour of some classes of women' (Gilman 1923: 735).[14] These are strong words. Her concern was that, in the cities in particular, women were showing an 'unmistakeable tendency to imitate the vices of men' (ibid.: 735). She chastised women for 'exhibitionism' or flaunting the body (Gilman 1963 [1935]). But she appeared to believe – or perhaps hope – that this was a temporary effect of rapid social change. As noted in the introduction to this book and as we will see in the chapters to come, these concerns have in fact echoed through time.

Conclusion

It has been my contention in this chapter that, far from taking flight from matters of the body to take shelter in the world of reason, early feminists brought an embodied health politics into being. Many were acutely aware from direct personal experience that mind–body dualism sanctioned patriarchy by permitting men to associate themselves with the positive and socially valued (the rational–mind–reason–health) and women with the negative and devalued (the irrational–body–emotion–illness). Arguing for women's inclusion in the world of reason alone would never have been enough to secure their liberation because this simply would have left negative perceptions of their 'defective' bodies intact. Physical and mental illness were presented as natural to women, but to many early feminists it was clear that their origins lay elsewhere. Showing that states of health arose from the social relations of society placed mind and body in contiguity. This embryonic sense of embodied health (involving a fusion of mind and body) held out the potential of a health activism that, if it was not yet able to undermine, could at least trouble the association of women with the negative and devalued (the natural–body–emotion–illness). Far from being an 'absent presence', health and the body were visibly at the heart of this simultaneously sociological and feminist thinking.

   This does not mean to say that the work of these women thinkers was without difficulty. One problem was the tendency to address their concerns to women of privilege. As noted earlier, Astell was strongly opposed to reform in the class structure and seemed only interested in a new future for women of means. Wollstonecraft was a supporter of the French Revolution and despised the aristocracy, so much so that she did not believe that aristocratic woman could ever be rehabilitated. But she gave relatively little attention to working-class women, directing the *Vindication of the Rights of Woman* to the wives of the new bourgeoisie whom she identified as the class possessing the most means to effect change since they had the most to gain. Martineau outwardly expressed her concern for reform in the lives of women from all social classes, writing at length, for example, about the dire conditions of working women's lives and the improvements that would benefit their health. However, her reformer's zeal has attracted criticism. For example, Deidre David remarks that from her home in Ambleside (in the Lake District area of England), she 'exercised woman's innate moral superiority through improvement of her lower-class neighbours by giving them weekly lectures on such matters as intemperance, terrifying her ruffianly audience into compliance by showing them pictures of a drunkard's stomach'! (1987: 55). It has been argued that Gilman's social evolutionary views made her blind to her own racism (Hill 1980). She maintained that there were 'deep, wide, lasting vital differences between the races' and feared that if not checked, the 'dwindling number of Americans' would be 'ruled over by a majority of conglomerate races', although she did remark that 'perhaps we should welcome our superseders, perhaps they will do better than we' in organising society (Gilman 1963 [1935]: 329). In discussing what she saw as the problems to society of the freeing of imported slaves, she took her observation that the 'African race' had 'with the advance of contact with our more advanced stage of evolution . . . made more progress in a few generations than any other race has ever done in the same time, except the Japanese' as proof that social evolution works, failing to see the racism and ethnocentrism in her argument (Gilman 1908: 80). Clearly, then, in common with many of their contemporaries, the legacy of these women thinkers on issues of class and 'race' is tarnished.
   Although several centuries passed between the work of Astell and Gilman, feminism was, so to speak, still very much finding its wings in the 1920s. This is why I have sought to emphasise that, in this fledgling journey, they were able to use health to *trouble* philosophical dualism, rather than, in any fundamental sense, to undermine it. Thus, while I have argued that they did not take flight from biology, it should be clear that their emphasis was nevertheless on the social. There is some sense of how a positive re-valuing of what is distinctive about women's bodies, such as their reproductive capacities, might advance their cause, for example, in Gilman's work. But it was changing *attitudes* towards women's bodies – such as those of the medical profession – that mattered. Consequently a full sense

of women's relationships *to* their bodies is underdeveloped. It could not be otherwise, because their politics was contingent upon keeping to the fore the argument that women's bodily oppression was social, not natural. As will be discussed in the chapters that follow, the particular form that the relationship between the natural and the social – or, what was to become known as sex and gender – has taken in research has been absolutely crucial to the way in which women's health has been understood.

2 Making connections
Feminism, sociology and health

Introduction

The previous chapter explored the ways in which early feminists were able to use the embodied experience of health and illness as a vehicle to trouble the dualisms that sustained patriarchal power. This placed mind and body in contiguity and held out the potential for an embodied health activism. The current chapter picks up these concerns as they were developed by feminists and others from around the mid-twentieth century through to the late 1970s and early 1980s.

The Second World War popularly is thought to have brought new opportunities for women with respect to employment and personal independence, including sexual freedom and greater bodily autonomy, although in effect this was only for a minority and was in any case short-lived (Caine 1997). Ideas of 'natural femininity' were to reassert themselves with a vengeance in the post-war period. The natural/social distinction that early feminists rallied against reached its twentieth-century height around this time. The marked tendency for the expanding discipline of sociology to absorb, rather than to challenge, this bi-polar social script motivated feminist sociologists and fellow travellers to craft a distinction between biological sex and social gender. A productive tension arose as sociological explanations for women's health were drawn towards the social and the wider body politic, while those of feminist health activists were equally, if not more, concerned with the individual experience of the reproductive or biological body.

The bi-polar social script

'Industrial capitalism' relied upon a relatively fixed and seemingly natural binary difference between man (employment-oriented, producer) and woman (home-based, consumer) (Bradley 2007; Fuat Firat 1994; Hennessy 2000). As Donald Lowe puts it, 'only in such a context does it make sense to see gender as a social script built upon bi-polar difference' (1995: 139). As noted in Chapter 1, the gender ideologies of any period are always 'in the

making' and, consequently, they are fissured, contested and open to oppositional formulations (Jordanova 1999; Poovey 1988), not least because of
local variability. The early decades of twentieth-century America, for
example, saw not only the emergence of the 'professional housewife' but
also the liberated flapper who so concerned Charlotte Perkins Gilman,
discussed in Chapter 1. It therefore would be wrong to portray the bi-
polar social script as hegemonic in form. This said, reflecting on her own
experience of growing up in 1940s and 1950s England, Harriet Bradley
remarks on how 'completely unchallenged and taken for granted [the] bi-
polar world of the sexes seemed' (2007: 16–17). And, as Elizabeth Roberts
discusses generally for the family lives of working-class women in the
north of England between the 1940s and the 1970s, 'however much attitudes
changed, changes in an institution as fundamental as the family were slow-
moving' (1995: 18). Thus as Roberts remarks, it is one of the ironies of
history that domestic ideology reached full flowering just at the time when
women's employment was being widely campaigned for. Evidently transformations in wider social attitudes often run ahead of changes in the actual
lives of the majority and the influence of established ideologies remains
strong. Women's magazines, for example, continued to endorse the overriding importance of marriage and the family during this period despite
women's growing labour force participation (Ferguson 1983). The trend
towards almost universal marriage that began in the 1920s lasted well into
the 1970s. Post-war Britons, for instance, broke all records as marriage
rates doubled for men and almost trebled for women aged in their twenties
between the 1940s and 1970s (Coleman 2000). Thus the male bread-winner
model remained culturally strong well into the 1970s (Davidoff 1995;
Tong 2007; Zweiniger-Bargielowska 2001a).

Consumerism was a vital instrument of women's domestication as the
production of mass commodities transformed the 'home-maker from a
home producer of goods to a purchaser of commodities' (Bradley 2007;
Matthaei 1982: 164; Pumphrey 1987). Even though they were presumed
to be natural experts when it came to consuming for the domestic realm
and for themselves, women's instinctive desire was not left alone; it still
needed to be directed towards the assortment of new goods on offer,
which ranged over the decades from electric irons, washing machines and
cleaning products, to 'as seen on TV' gadgets (Clarke 2000; Roberts 1995).
For example, the British Ideal Home Exhibitions did not simply showcase
goods; they educated women in homemaking with demonstrations and
advice in the new science and vocation of the domestic (Ryan 2000). The
exhibitions, the first in 1908 (and, interestingly, subject to suffragette
protest), 'presented a vision of stable femininity and peaceful domesticity'
(ibid.: 10). For example, an advertisement in the *Daily Mail* newspaper
(which sponsors the exhibitions to this day) implied that the vision of the
ideal wife–ideal home life set before young men was so dazzling that they
could be moved to propose to their girlfriends (ibid.). The implication no

doubt was that an ideal home and a husband in one fell swoop was just too much for most women to resist.

It was within this context that feminist research on health began to take shape. Its resulting form grew out of the tensions and breakthroughs in its relationship with mainstream sociology and with activist feminism. As recently as the late 1960s, 'neither the topic of women, nor the existence of women as sociologists were apparent' (Delamont 2003: 16). Barbara Laslett and Barrie Thorne (1997) draw on Dorothy Smith's (1974) notion of a 'bifurcated consciousness' to depict the experiences of women who entered sociology in the late 1960s and early 1970s: on the one hand, they were committed to their discipline; on the other, they were patently aware that there was a yawning gap between their experiences as women and the frameworks that sociology provided to explain them. Change, of course, did not come at all easy (see, for example, Banks 1999; Deem 1996; Evans 2003; Oakley 1974a). One of the most pressing problems was the uncritical reproduction of the bi-polar social script within the discipline.

The notion of social roles took off in the 1950s, particularly in the United States where structural functionalism was in the ascendancy (e.g. Parsons and Bales 1956). As befitted the time, appropriate male/female roles – respectively instrumental and expressive in form – were consonant with biological sex and complementary to each other. Auguste Comte – who coined the term sociology – inaugurated this line of thought in the mid-nineteenth century with his assertion that, with their emotional and affective natures, women are less human than men. In his own words, woman is unfit 'for the continuousness and intensity of mental labour, either from the intrinsic weakness of her reason or from her more lively moral and physical sensibility, which are hostile to scientific abstraction and concentration' (Comte 1830–42: 269). Consequently, woman's place in the family – the basic unit of social life – is naturally subordinate, where her role is to modify 'the cold and rough reason that is distinctive of man' (ibid.: 269). Émile Durkheim (1968 [1893]; 1970 [1897]) continued this theme, often directly replicating Comte's expression, with the claim that women are asocial beings who have been left behind in a state of nature. For Durkheim, the so-called sexual division of labour is doubly determined: by reference to nature (the differential natures of men and women) and through the social functions that these natural differences serve (Lehmann 1994).

The legacy of Comte, Durkheim and others was taken forward into empirical sociology during the 1960s and 1970s and beyond, most notably in research on the family, the very domain that was high in the consciousness of the new generation of women sociologists. For example, in his exegesis, William Goode was aware that very little of the 'sexual division of labour' is required by 'the biological peculiarities of the two sexes' and that, more often than not, it is at heart unequal, given that male tasks, whatever they may be, are 'defined as more honorific' (1964: 70). But it seemed that there was little that could be done about this, since it was what society in general, and the family in particular, demanded. It was in response to this ascription that Ann Oakley and others declared the division of labour by sex to be a myth, imported into sociology from without. Oakley observed that, if the function of myth generally is to maintain the status quo, then 'the sociologist overtly declares this to be part of "his" theoretical enterprise' (Oakley 1974b: 178). Ostensibly value-free, 'the sociological argument translates as, the oppression of women is convenient, whilst their liberation would be inconvenient: a disruptive and destructive force' (ibid.: 182–3). Thus sociology ends up confirming that women's unpaid labour as child-rearers, housewives and the servants of men is essential to the smooth running of society. As Betty Freidan put it, 'at a time of great change for women, at a time when education, science and social science should have helped women bridge the change, functionalism transformed "what is", or "what was", to "what should be"' (1963: 120). The host of responsibilities heaped upon women included liability for how children turn out. Mothering became increasingly exacting work at this time as influential theories such as that of John Bowlby (1951) drew attention to the perceived ill-effects of 'maternal deprivation' in early childhood (Thane 1994). Goode (1964) not only placed the socialisation of children but also their achievements in life squarely on their mother's shoulders, debating, for example, on the effect of women 'going out to work'. The replication of wider gender ideology in terms of the pecking order in the family is more than apparent in his use of language: marriage is defined in terms of the husband and his wife (not husband and wife, and certainly not the wife and her husband).

The strong fit between the structural functionalist orthodoxy and male domination of the sociological agenda not only kept critical reflection on 'gender divisions' out of the frame, but also related topics of interest to women. Thus, Oakley (1974a) struggled to get her research on housework taken seriously. Stevi Jackson recounts that, when as a postgraduate she expressed an interest in the study of sexuality, 'most established academics responded either with incomprehension or with ribald and sexist innuendo' (1999: 8).[1] The reasons why health and illness were not on the sociological agenda are easy to discern. Parsons and others had simply carried forward what had gone before. As discussed at the start of Chapter 1, the neglect of health and the body did not simply flow from philosophical dualism but from the related flight from all that was female-defined. Since women were equated with an unruly and defective body – that is, with illness – to have drawn health and illness into the sociological fold would have risked casting it in decidedly feminine or female terms. To put it simplistically, if men could transcend biology – something that was very important to the sociology of the time – women could not. As Olive Banks reflected, the reproductive or biological determinism in the theories of Parsons and others 'ruled out any possibility of change favourable to women' (1999: 406). It therefore made perfect sense for feminists to counter with two claims: first, that women are no more (or less) determined by their biology than are men; and, second, that the image of women's biology that patriarchy presents to the world is grossly misconstrued. From these two claims it was possible to deduce that women's oppression is socially caused, rather than biologically given. The basis for this argument was the powerful distinction between sex (biology) and gender (social).

Sex and gender

As was discussed in Chapter 1, although the concept of 'gender' itself was not yet in circulation, its spirit was evident in embodied health politics at least as far back as the late seventeenth century. New momentum came in the 1920s and 1930s with Margaret Mead's anthropological studies of South Seas cultures. From her research Mead deduced that 'socially defined sex differences ... obviously cannot be true for all humanity – or the people over the mountain would not be able to do it all in the exactly opposite fashion'. But she questioned whether, notwithstanding its variable form, the tendency to mould different qualities or traits onto different biological bodies might be a universal phenomenon or, as she put it, a superstructure (Mead 1971 [1950]: 32). In other words, even though it expresses itself differently by time and place, is the division a kind of *must* for society? Would it always be with us?

The actual term 'gender' initially found expression in psychiatry. Based on his work with intersexed patients and transsexuals, Robert Stoller argued that :

> while *sex* and *gender* seem to common sense to be practically synony-mous, and in everyday life to be inextricably bound together, [the two realms] are not at all inevitably bound in anything like a one-to-one relationship, but may each go in its independent way.
>
> (Stoller 1968: ix, emphasis original)

Stoller's point was not that biology has no role, but rather that its 'weaker qualities' are hidden by what he saw as the overwhelming effects of gender socialisation. Sexologist John Money was far less circumspect about biology's influence. His observation that children whose chromosomal sex failed to match their external genitalia developed, as he put it, a gender identity that was appropriate to their gender socialisation suggested to him that, in some cases, gender was so arbitrary that it might even be contrary to physiology.

A case initially described by Money in the early 1970s was, sadly, to become the subject of enduring debate. Physicians decided that an infant boy born in 1965, whose penis had been accidentally ablated flush to the abdominal wall during circumcision, would be unable to develop a 'normal' male identity and that, following plastic surgery, should be brought up as a girl. Money explained: 'we gave the parents confidence' that their child 'could be expected to differentiate a female gender identity, in agreement with the sex of her rearing' (Money and Ehrhardt 1972: 119). The case was of particular interest to the scientific community because the child, Bruce Reimer, renamed Brenda, had an identical twin brother, Brian. Money described how Brenda grew up to be a 'typical girl' and Brian, a 'typical boy'. As Suzanne Kessler puts it, 'the case was cited as proof of the plasticity of gender and appeared to have struck a mighty blow to biological determinism' (1998: 6). However, the passage of time was to throw Money's assertions – as well as his credibility – into serious doubt. Milton Diamond located Reimer, whom Money claimed had been 'lost to follow-up' many years on and discovered that he had never accepted a female gender identity and had in fact undergone surgery to convert 'back' to a male with the chosen name of David (Diamond and Sigmundson 1997; and see Colapinto 2000). A series of personal crises and misfortunes, including the suicide of his brother Brian, culminated in David taking his own life in 2004. Intersex and sex reassignment surgery continue to be important points of reference in the discussion of the sex (biology) and gender (social) distinction. The important point at this juncture is that this was the environment within which sociological and feminist research on gender and health developed.

Ann Oakley argued that:

> 'sex' is a word that refers to the biological differences between male and female: the visible difference in genitalia, the related difference in procreative function. 'Gender' however is a matter of culture: it refers to the social classification into the 'masculine' and 'feminine'.
>
> (1972: 16)

This formulation provided the essential challenge to the bi-polar script within academic sociology. The point of Oakley's argument was not that sex and gender bear no relationship to each other, but rather that 'the aura of naturalness and inevitability that surrounds gender-differentiation in modern society comes [. . .] from the beliefs people hold about it' (ibid.: 189), and not from biology. This resonated widely within the emerging feminist sociology of the time. For example, Maren Lockwood Carden remarked that the 'new feminists' were basing their argument for equality upon 'the belief that the biologically derived differences between the sexes are relatively minor and that a vast inequitable system has been built upon the assumption that such differences are basic and major' (1974: 11). As we will see in Chapter 3, much of this literature was framed in terms of individual roles and role change. However, Gayle Rubin drew attention to the wider social system within which the biological and social relate to each other. Thus she made clear that, 'sex/gender systems are not ahistorical emanations of the human mind; they are products of historical human activity' (Rubin 1975: 204), that is, they are situated in time and place. For mid-twentieth-century women, the place of their lives was principally the home and, as we have seen, the predominant sociological theory of the time only served to reinforce this.

Although the potential of the sex/gender distinction to illuminate the harms to women's bodies and their health shines out when looking back, it was far from easy for the new generation of female sociologists to bring it to light at the time. The women's movement was drawing increasingly vocal attention to women's health-related oppression, but this filtered relatively slowly into academia. Health lagged behind other topics of greater interest to the new generation of feminist sociologists such as work and industry, social stratification, and the family (although some of this did have health implications). The newly developing area of medical sociology, in its turn, was slow to take an interest in gender and, when it did, was often more concerned with using women's experience of ill health or of health care as a resource to explore broader sociological issues and with re-working existing frameworks to accommodate women than with developing new frameworks that would speak *for* them.

The women's health movement

The distinction between feminist activists and feminist academics is somewhat artificial since, from the start, activists published in academic collections and many academic feminists were either personally engaged in the women's movement or they envisaged that their research would have a direct influence upon it. Nonetheless, in its early development, the women's movement 'remained fundamentally political and insulated from scholarly focus' (Olesen and Lewin 1985: 9). Writing about her first encounter with feminism through political resistance to the Vietnam War and the founding of 'Bread and Roses' (a socialist-feminist women's group on the US East Coast), Barrie Thorne (1997) explains that those who entered the field of sociology and the women's liberation movement more or less in tandem found that, while the two worlds sometimes met with thrilling resonance, they also collided.

Although women's testimonies bear witness to unprecedented and exhilarating change for the better in many women's lives, the women's movement defies easy description, particularly with respect to its origins. In the thick of it, Germaine Greer (1971) wrote that we can only speculate as to its causes. It is clear in retrospect that the term 'women's movement' gives deceptive coherence to a movement that was diverse and changing. It was collective, in the sense that all women to varying degrees bore witness to at least the promise of sweeping social and political change, but it was also highly piecemeal, existing in the scores of local activist groups and networks that sprang up in response to a jigsaw of specific concerns, such as women's health. This amoebic quality and the 'infinite variety of groups, strategies and organisations' involved (Freeman 1973: 795) posed difficulties for feminist sociologists of the time as they sought to understand its likely future. Thus, writing in the *American Journal of Sociology*, Jo Freeman (1973) referred to the lack of regard for wider institutional change in the thousands of virtually independent 'sister chapters' around the US – many based around friendship groups and fairly homogenous in terms of social class, age, and ethnicity – which were mainly concerned with personal change using instruments such as the consciousness-raising group.

Broadly speaking, the women's movement was influenced by the radical politics of the US civil rights movement and Left politics (in Britain and elsewhere in Europe) (Carden 1974; Freeman 1973; Rowbotham 1972, 2000). The civil rights movement sent the clear message that 'if collective action could destroy racial segregation, which was based on the belief in white superiority, why couldn't women challenge ideas about female inferiority?' (Rosen 2000: 59). In Britain, equal pay strikes of the 1960s and the 'wages for housework' campaign highlighted class issues and the relationship between the women's movement and the political left. The idea of wages for housework, which was highly debated within the women's movement, threw the link between socialism and feminism into particular relief. The argument went that, if housework is economically important insofar as it involves the production and reproduction of commodities for capitalism; that is, the maintenance of husbands and children, as well as the woman herself for the workforce, then it generates surplus value and women deserve a wage (see Dalla Costa and James 1995 [1972]; Gardiner 1976; Malos 1995). However, as discussed at the start of the chapter, for most women, the new world that beckoned, such as the unprecedented new freedoms in employment and in the control of fertility, stopped resolutely at their kitchen or bedroom door. Betty Freidan's *The Feminist Mystique* (1963) in the US and Hannah Gavron's *The Captive Wife* (1966) in Britain awakened feminist concerns about women's homemaker roles that had been slumbering since at least the 1940s. As noted earlier, there was a large gap between the fetishised femininity of post-war domesticity (Coote and Campbell 1987) and its hidden exploitation, which was alive and well in most women's own homes, and the wider cultural and political discontent that Greer (1971) and others exhorted women to prize. It was this gap that was to provoke the eponymous slogan: 'the personal is political'.

As Sandra Morgen makes clear in her history of the women's health movement in the US, even though it was 'always hewed to its local beginnings', personal involvement and the knowledge that there were others who were equally engaged, generated the strong feeling that the movement was palpable, embodied, real (Morgen 2002: 11). 'Members of women's health organisations believed that they were responding to, as well as nourishing, an inexorable force' (ibid.: 40). To give some sense of the scope and reach of the movement, it is estimated that, by the early 1970s, there were at least 1,000 organisations engaged in some form of women's health activism and over 150 free clinics providing a range of services, such as pregnancy testing, abortion (or abortion referrals), gynaecological services and contraception in the US (Morgen 2002; Ruzek 1978).[2] The wealth of experiential data that poured forth highlighted two crucial things: the negative consequences of male medical control of the female body and the ability of women to seize this control in their own interests. Forty or so years on, it can be difficult to appreciate the radical nature of this realisation. Yet even a cursory glance at the literature of the time makes it abundantly clear. The archives of the influential Boston Women's Health Book Collective, for example, provide compelling evidence of the 'life changing effect' for women of finding out about their bodies and their needs. Formed in 1969 in Massachusetts, the Collective grew out of a Boston workshop on 'women and their bodies'. As they shared their experiences, many for the very first time, the women began to appreciate that their anger and frustration towards specific doctors and towards the 'medical maze' in general, was shared. These 'doctor stories' were the springboard for a series of local courses on women's health. The recognition that 'body education' was liberation prompted the founders to write *Our Bodies, Ourselves* (1978), which went on to become a worldwide best selling book, translated and adapted into twenty languages (Davis 2002a). First published commercially in 1973 and currently in its eleventh edition, the book is widely credited with 'changing the landscape of women's healthcare in the United States and around the world' (Morgen 2002: 5; see also Davis 2002a; 2007b).[3]

Towards the end of the 1970s, Claudia Dreifus explicitly used the term 'health feminism', which she defined as a movement of women 'including housewives, mothers, students, lesbians, socialists, herbalists', all united in 'their common femaleness, their distrust of organised medicine' (1978: xxv). The angry responses that practices such as showing women how to use a speculum for vaginal self-examination provoked from established medicine were witnessed in doctors' surgeries across the US, as well as publicly. In 1972, activist Carol Downer was arrested, went to trial, and was later acquitted, for practising medicine without a licence. The catalyst was the observation by an undercover policewoman of her use of yoghurt to treat a woman's vaginal yeast infection at an evening meeting of the Los Angeles Feminist Health Centre. Columnist Barbara Seaman's (1995 [1969]) exposé of the health risks posed by the oral contraceptive pill shook the US medical establishment and led, in 1970, to the Senate hearings that eventually mandated the inclusion of health warnings on all prescription drugs, and helped to establish the principle of informed consent.

In Britain, access free of charge and the iconic status of the National Health Service, 'which symbolised the vision of a collectivist society', meant that most feminists took it for granted that they should seek to transform the system from within (Doyal 2006: 151; Pringle 1998). A network of community well woman clinics were set up during the late 1970s and early 1980s and the Workers' Educational Association played (and continues to play) a key role in promoting women's health education (Black and Ong 1986). The wider link between the women's movement and health activism in Britain is evident in a range of publications from the 1970s. For example, *Spare Rib. A Women's Liberation Magazine*, carried a range of articles that, like the Boston Women's Health Book Collective, showed women how to 'bring knowledge of their bodies back to themselves'. Two collections of articles: *The Spare Rib Reader* (Rowe 1982), covering the period 1972–78, and *Women's Health. A Spare Rib Reader* (O'Sullivan 1987), covering 1970 to around the mid-1980s, address topics as wide ranging as menstruation, abortion, breast cancer, radical midwifery, toxic shock syndrome, mental ill health and health hazards at work.

The body/body politic problem

Grass roots health activism provided the essential evidence for what feminists had been arguing for centuries; that women's malaise was socially produced rather than rooted in their inferior biology. It is instructive to note that in the US, Carol Downer's first public cervical self-examination is generally seen as the event that, more than any other, transformed health and body issues into a separate movement (Morgen 2002; Ruzek 1978). This is highly symbolic of the wider focus of the movement on the reproductive body or, more accurately, aspects of the reproductive body. And herein lay some dangers. As Lynda Birke puts it, 'women have long been subject to medical ideologies that construct us as little more than wombs on legs, which a feminist focus on reproduction does not always challenge' (1999: 12). Susan Reverby remarks that, even at the time, 'I never thought looking through a plastic speculum was a way to see power' (Bell and Reverby 2005: 436). She worried that, no matter how much she spoke about the bigger picture, women 'seemed only to focus on their own bodies' (ibid.: 436). Equally, Ellen Frankfort (1972) pointed out that, important though they were, doctors, hospitals and drug companies were not going to be affected by having small groups of women learning how to examine their cervixes or how to extract their menstrual periods. She wanted women to organise around the institutions where the power lay.

Susan Bell and Susan Reverby encapsulate this as the body/body politic problem: how to connect individual body concerns with the wider structures of oppression. They draw parallels with today's *Vagina Monologues* (Ensler 2001). While recognising the individual transformative potential of the play, they worry whether it 're-instates women's problems in our bodies, indeed in our vaginas alone' (Bell and Reverby 2005: 438). In the 1970s, as now, the focus on individual experience or 'self-help' in relation to the 'sexual organs' has a troubling resemblance to the medical focus on women's distinctive 'body parts'. As Susan Bell discusses with respect to her contribution to the 1984 revision of *Our Bodies, Ourselves*, by repeating the 'standard logic and terms presented in leading medical texts' about matters such as menstruation, the book tended unwittingly to conform to medical images of women's bodies at the same time as it tried to challenge them (Bell 1994: 12). As well as fixing fragmented medical imagery in women's imagination in the manner later described by Emily Martin (1987), rather ironically, this 'looking inside' part paved the way for women's general acceptance of the technologisation of birth, such as ultrasound imaging (Kuhlmann forthcoming). I say 'ironically' because, as discussed in Chapter 4, the medicalisation of birth became an abiding concern.

To sum up the argument so far, the women's health movement was one part in a constellation of factors – although possibly the guiding star – that shaped how the sex/gender distinction came to be used in the study of women's health. As we have seen, the body/body politic problem (Bell and Reverby 2005) encapsulated the tensions between activism, which stressed the personal (as political), and the sociological will to analyse wider social oppression or the body politic. The sex/gender distinction as articulated by Oakley (1972) and others had drawn academic feminism towards the social and pulled it away from the biological. Yet, with its focus on the distinctive female reproductive body, it seemed to be the biological that mattered to much of the women's health movement, albeit with a vital twist since women's liberation lay in a positive revaluing of women's biological bodies (see further discussion in Chapter 3). As I will now go on to discuss, this focus was also at variance with the dominant academic agenda where, in the early development of the sociology of gender and medical sociology, it was the social (not the biological) that mattered most.

Gender, the social and medical sociology

Medical sociologists[4] shared a common disciplinary project with feminists generally, which was to distinguish the biological from the social, which dovetailed – at least in theory – with the sex/gender problematic. From the vantage of medical sociology, this involved differentiating its own 'social' approach to health and illness from the medical profession's focus on the biological body. For example, in his landmark publication *Profession of Medicine*, Eliot Freidson (1970) proposed that illness could be thought of as a biological or physical state that exists independently of human knowledge and evaluation and also as a social state that is shaped by these self-same factors. Illness as a *physical* state, he argued, is the province of medicine, while health as a *social* state is the topic of the new discipline of medical sociology. By taking on this distinction, sociologists were carving out an intellectual domain all of their own (Strong 1979). The social imperialism and consequent disembodied approach that was to characterise medical sociology for some time was a legacy of the strong belief of the nineteenth-century 'founding fathers' that social interaction – the principal object of enquiry – could never be reduced to biology or physiology, as already discussed in Chapter 1.

The strong conceptual affinity between the new wave of post-Second-World-War feminism and early medical sociology was coupled with a shared experience of exclusion. Much in the manner that feminism was rebuffed by 'malestream' academia, the sociology of health and illness traditionally has been undervalued by wider sociology. The lukewarm reception in sociology departments was related to the higher regard given to labour markets, social divisions and religion than to health and illness, which customarily was seen as applied (many of its practitioners worked in settings concerned with the training of health care providers, which remains the case today) and therefore of low status. No doubt its purportedly feminine or female subject matter – namely, the body and caring work – only added to this. But the experience of common problems is not bound to result in unity of purpose. Sara Delamont (2003) is right to note that the sociology of health and illness has been transformed by feminism, but the two academic fields are more appropriately described – historically and today – as parallel rather than integrated projects. If we go back to the early days of medical sociology in the 1960s and 1970s, it is clear that, even though 'women's issues' were gaining a foot-hold, the malestream agenda that dominated wider sociology had a firm grip.

Oftentimes it was not women qua women than mattered to researchers; they were simply convenient respondents. For example, George Brown and his female collaborator Tirril Harris appear initially to have chosen to research women in their influential study, the *Social Origins of Depression*, more for practical reasons than for any commitment to the social oppression that provoked women's much higher rates of mental ill health. They relate that since large-scale research can be financially prohibitive, 'one way to reduce its costs was to study women only, as they probably suffer from depression more often than men' (Brown and Harris 1978: 22). Moreover, women were ready subjects at the behest of these researchers. Thus, 'we would need to approach only half as many women as men to obtain the same number with depressive disorders' (ibid.: 22). 'It also seemed likely', they continue, 'that women, who are more often at home during the day, would be more willing to agree to see us for several hours, the time we needed to collect our material' (ibid.: 22).

Broadly speaking, we can identify three closely related problems in medical sociology of the time. First, was the inclination to treat women's experience as a topic to be 'added in' to the existing canon, that is, to fashion a 'gender awareness' rather than to overhaul existing theory to account fully for women's health-related experience. Second, was the tendency to use women's experience of health care primarily as a resource to explore broader sociological concerns. Third, was the propensity to use male experience as the benchmark or 'gold standard' for interpreting the experience of women.

There were indications that sociology generally was becoming more 'gender aware' during the 1970s and early 1980s. This was evident in criticisms of existing approaches, such as the annotated bibliography of the British Sociological Association (BSA), *Sociology Without Sexism* (1977), as well as in the deliberations on the 'state of the field' and the discipline's future. For example, in their introduction to a collection marking the thirtieth anniversary of the BSA, Philip Abrams and colleagues wrote that 'the feminist intervention in sociology has been a particularly important one because it has been able to show how one-sided the theories and researches of many sociologists – both male and female – have been hitherto' (1981: 3). Although positive in tone, the editors' support is nonetheless circumscribed, since their agenda appears to extend only to making women 'sociologically visible' and to the 'capacity of sociology informed by feminist thought to broaden the range of sociological concerns' (ibid.: 9). Clearly this is not a sociology *for* women but a sociology informed by 'women's issues'. Similarly, in *Recent British Sociology*, John Eldridge (1980) drew readers' attention to the neglect of 'gender differences' in areas such as community studies and industrial sociology. He remarked that the discipline was at risk of becoming a 'sociology of this and that' – the sociology *of* industry, the sociology *of* sex and gender, and so on; that is, a sociology of sub-divisions. Despite this, Eldridge was optimistic that the 'sociological imagination', a term coined by C. Wright Mills (1975 [1959]), offered a way forward.[5] Yet, despite including an indicative bibliography on 'sex, gender and generation', Eldridge failed to extend his remarks about the lack of attention to women and gender to any sustained analysis of the state of the field. Rather his discussion was limited to pre-existing areas such as economic life, criminology, education and religion.

Although North American and British medical sociology texts, collections and research articles from the 1970s contain a smattering of references to women and several reports of research on women's health or health care, almost without exception here, too, it is women as a topic that interests authors, rather than a feminist interpretation of women's experience. As might be expected, the tendency to use women's experience of ill health or of health care as a resource to explore broader sociological concerns is most apparent in texts, chapters in edited collections and articles by male authors. For example, William Rosengren and Spencer DeVault were interested in how time and space 'define, legitimate, sanction and handle expressions of pain' in the obstetric hospital (1978: 202). They were squarely focused on how organisations structure social action and pay little or no attention to the hospital as a hierarchical organisation that attributes power to men, or to the problems that this might pose for women in childbirth. However, female authors were not immune to these problems either. Two well-known research articles serve to illustrate this.

In 'K is mentally ill', Dorothy Smith (1978) was interested in accounts of mental illness. This was part of the wider, and at the time controversial, sociological argument that mental illness is a form of escape from a difficult social reality, rather than, as the conventional medical model would have it, a malfunctioning of the brain (see, for example, Scheff 1966). In her article Smith is concerned with the conceptual work or meaning making that K's friends – all young undergraduate students – engage in as they move towards the definition of her behaviour as an anomaly rather than 'just' deviations from a norm or social rule. As sociological interpreter, Smith is also interested in whether an alternative reading 'of the goings on could be drawn' (Smith 1978: 25). She demonstrates the steps by which K's friends come to the conclusion that she is mentally ill and suggests an alternative reading, which is that K was experiencing the 'freezing-out process' that can happen in a relationship between three friends (ibid.: 25). It is interesting that while Smith does not privilege one interpretation over another – since she stresses that the account can be read for the 'mental illness effect' (ibid.: 26) or in terms of her alternative 'freezing out effect' – a possible 'gender effect' is not considered, despite some 'clues' that it is K's experience as a woman that may matter most. Thus, K's friends make reference to problems with young men, that she was terrified of anyone getting near to her, especially men; to 'definite food-fads'; and to excessive exercising. While these aspects need not point to mental illness any more than Smith's interpretation of 'freezing out' does, they do signal the possibility of personal problems that relate to the experience of young womanhood, which is not considered.

A second illustration comes from Joan Emerson's well-known (1970) analysis of gynaecological examinations. Emerson's purpose was to ground empirically sociologists Peter Berger and Thomas Luckmann's (1966) theoretical notion of the 'social construction of reality', which, at the time, was growing in popularity as a counter to the structural functionalist orthodoxy, referred to earlier. Emerson's aim was to take observations of a 'concrete situation [. . .] to show how reality is embodied in routines and reaffirmed in social interaction' (1970: 75). The gynaecological examination was chosen, first because it was an excellent example of multiple contradictory definitions of reality and, second, because participants' incapacity to perform appropriately was a substantial threat to sustaining the dominant reality of the situation as 'medical' rather than 'sexual'. Emerson details how the dominant medical reality is achieved, drawing on observational data from seventy-five examinations conducted by male physicians. She found that since they are immersed in a medical world that is routine to them, medical staff assume the main responsibility for a credible performance, guiding the patient to adopt a nonchalant, matter of fact pose and making it clear that their own interest is simply technical. Yet at the same time, the physician must also, to some extent, acknowledge the patient as a person. Counter-definitions of reality therefore enter the scene. These are dealt with by pulling the medical definition back in – for example, by drawing attention to the clinical environment, by the use of special language that bypasses sexual imagery, through the presence of a nurse as a chaperone, and so on. As Emerson put it, 'the self must be eclipsed in order to sustain the definition that the doctor is working on a technical object and not a person' (ibid.: 83).

Health activist Carol Downer, discussed earlier, took exception to this account, remarking that, while Emerson's study concerns women's health and focuses on male (doctor)–female (patient) interaction, it singularly neglects to question the appropriateness of this way of examining women's genitals and to consider why 'parties are willing to go through this charade'; and it fails to account for the embarrassment and uneasiness that was observed (Downer 1972). In Downer's opinion, this 'social myopia' seriously inhibits feminist understanding. There are, she asserts, far more penetrating questions to be asked, such as: why must women be examined by male physicians at all? It is clear then that female sociologists' attempts to take issues that concern women as case studies for the development of wider sociological agendas were unlikely to meet with the unqualified approval of feminist activists outside the academy. There is still a tendency today for writers on women's health care to read a feminist critique into Emerson's analysis (see, for example, Sandelowski 1981: 152–4). Although less theoretically sophisticated, by identifying gynaecology as one of the 'forces committed to maintaining traditional sex-role stereotypes, in the interest of men and from a male perspective' Diana Scully and Pauline Bart's analysis of images of women in gynaecology textbooks over the period 1943–72 was more radical in intent (1973: 1045; see also Scully 2003).

In early medical sociology texts that discuss topics such as doctor–patient interaction, the experience of illness and health status differences, the focus more often than not is upon the 'generic male' (reinforced by the use of the male pronoun to refer to both patients and doctors). There is little or no discussion of *why* male/female differences exist, and certainly no recourse to gender inequality in explanation. Even topics that on the face of it seem to call out for critical discussion in these terms, such as nursing, receive no such attention.[6] In the preface to his 1970 text, for example, Robert Wilson relates that human health is 'a topic both of inherent interest to the curious sociologist and of compelling pragmatic importance to all who care about man's ability to live to capacity' (1970: 28). And, indeed, it is to 'generic man' that the text is addressed. So, in illustrating where patient–practitioner relationships 'go wrong', Wilson remarks that 'one of the familiar difficulties for male physicians is the reluctance of women in many traditional cultures to be examined and treated if this involves intimate access to the body' (ibid.: 28). Clearly, the difficulty as presented here is for the male doctor, not the female patient, and no thought is given to the possibility that female practitioners might alleviate the 'problem'.

Although male/female comparisons appear in places in a number of early medical sociology texts, typically under the rubric of 'social epidemiology' (for example in discussions of differential patterns of illness and life expectancy), generally speaking, this is framed in terms of deviation from a male 'gold standard'. For example, David Mechanic comes to the conclusion that much of the female 'excess' in morbidity (in comparison to men) probably reflects women's tendency to report more 'subjective symptoms' (compared to men). Thus he reports that 'while it is difficult to support the argument that women have more illness than men, apparently they feel or express more subjective distress of all kinds' (Mechanic 1978: 188). The intent to explain women's difference *from* men, rather than to think in terms of how men and women might differ *from each other*, is apparent in Mechanic's failure to at least consider the possibility that statistics might reflect the fact that men are less likely to 'feel or express' their real distress. Evidently, gendered responses are the prerogative of women, while men are the 'objective' ungendered benchmark in the debate (that is, gender has no bearing on their experience). This point notwithstanding, it is important to note that at least two early collections of articles did reproduce journal articles that were instrumental in taking feminist research on gender and health forward, and were to become landmark debates: Constance Nathanson's 'Sex, illness and medical care: a review of data, theory, and method' (in Albrecht and Higgins 1979) and Ingrid Waldron's 'Why do women live longer than men?' (in Mechanic 1980).

Some collections explicitly cite feminism's contribution to the field. For example, in the introduction to the edited collection *Health Care and Health Knowledge*, Robert Dingwall, Christian Heath, Margaret Reid and Margaret Stacey point out that 'some sociologists have found themselves drawn into an examination of medical encounters' through their sympathies with the feminist movement (1977: 10). Perhaps this inclusion reflects the combination of female and male editors. Certainly, women authors appear to be poised on the brink of finding a feminist voice during the 1970s. But, equally, they seem reluctant, or unable, to divest themselves of the theoretical trappings of conventional sociological understandings. For example, Alan Davis and Gordon Horobin's *Medical Encounters* (1977), an edited collection of sociologists' accounts of their own experiences of ill health, includes several chapters by women. Ann Holohan, Nicky Hart, Jean Comaroff and Sally Macintyre (the latter with David Oldman), for example, all make some reference to gender politics in their individual chapters. But in each case, this is fleeting and underdeveloped as a way of interpreting their experience. There were glimmers of the more developed feminist sociology of health that was still off on the horizon. For example, Jean Comaroff advances sociological knowledge – in this instance, what she terms the social and conceptual ambiguities of pregnancy – and also provides pragmatic insight into how women cope while in hospital. She documents two 'models of childbirth' – male/abnormal, female/normal-natural (see also Chapter 5) – that co-exist in the clinic and reveals how both may be drawn upon by women to impose 'systematic conceptual clarity' on their pregnancy as a 'transitional social condition', either by defining themselves as primarily healthy, primarily ill, or by confronting the 'ambiguities of their condition in largely situational terms' (Comaroff 1977: 131).

It was not until the 1980s that any sustained attention was given to feminist interpretations of women's experience in general medical sociology texts. For example, Peter Conrad and Rochelle Kern's (1981) *The Sociology of Health and Illness* contained a section entitled 'racism and sexism in medicine'. By the end of the decade, Margaret Stacey wrote directly 'as a woman and as a feminist' in *The Sociology of Health and Healing* (1988: xiii). But, lest it should be seen simply as a relic of the (not too distant) past, it should be pointed out that myopia to feminism lives on. Uta Gerhardt's (1989) intellectual and political history of medical sociology makes no reference to the contribution of feminism, nor does Samuel Bloom's more recent chronicle, *The Word as Scalpel* (2002), which focuses mainly on the United States.[7]

Conclusion

To the extent that they sit outside or on the margins of a wider feminist theoretical analysis of the social relations of gender, issues of heath are extremely vulnerable to co-optation and the loss of their critical feminist edge. In this chapter I have argued that early academic research on women's health was shaped by a constellation of factors that orbited the powerful sex (biology)/(social) gender distinction. This included feminist activism, which provided powerful grass roots evidence of women's health-related oppression and of the potential for change but nonetheless troubled some in its tendency to (re)turn attention to the individual reproductive body. It also included medical sociology, which was fervently interested in the social dimensions of health and illness but circumscribed women's health concerns by containing it within its own existing conceptual space. As I now go on to discuss in Chapter 3, research on health began to pull in two directions: towards the biological or towards the social. The latter was the acceptable face of sociological research on women's health by far. It dovetailed with the emphasis on the social within medical sociology and, precisely because it did not inflict undue damage upon the agenda as currently organised, it was more palatable to, and accommodating of, male sociologists and others working on health issues. It also fit the wider agenda of political liberalism, or 'equality feminism' where the object is economic, legal and social parity with men and biological difference should not matter.

It was not that more radical political alternatives were unavailable. As discussed earlier, a more radical feminist health activism was very influential outside the academy. This had the merit of being far less liable to incorporation and containment than liberal feminism but for this very reason was unlikely to find a voice within the academy in the first place. During the late 1970s and early 1980s, Marxism was advocated as a critical alternative to the structural functionalist orthodoxy within sociology, especially in Europe (see, for example, Banks 1970; Bottomore 1975; Bottomore and Goode 1983). This does not mean to say that feminists writing about women's health were neglectful of the wider political economy. For example, Lesley Doyal emphasised that any analysis of medicine and its treatment of women, had to be placed within a 'broader feminist critique of capitalist society' (1979: 237). But, more generally speaking, feminists working within Marxism or taking a political economy approach were as likely as radical feminists to be shunned and excluded by the male academic establishment. Although they may have found their political home within Marxism, they faced serious problems of containment by their brethren, many of whom argued that feminism was 'at best less important than class conflict and at worst divisive of the working class' (Hartmann 1981: 2; see also Delphy 1984). Arguably mid- to late-twentieth-century Marxist social science was no less guilty of reproducing the myths of patriarchy than was structural functionalism. For these reasons, both radical and Marxist or materialist feminism were less likely to find a place in the mainstream of feminist research on health and medicine than was liberal feminism, which was a far more palatable feminist 'brand' for the academy.

For these reasons liberal feminism became the acceptable and visible face of feminist sociological research on health and illness in the 1970s and early 1980s, but with radical feminism and Marxist or materialist feminism ever present as critical alternatives. The two chapters that follow explore two contrasting traditions that emerged during the 1970s: the more establishment-friendly 'liberal or equality feminism' and the more critical 'radical or difference feminism', and the lasting agenda that they set for future feminist sociological research on health and illness.

3 Women and health status

Introduction

The distinction between sex (biology) and gender (social) has been a conceptual treasure trove for research on health, but one that nevertheless has harboured problems. The foremost of these has been the tendency to draw research in one of two directions. One strand of research has stressed women's parity with men, played down biological difference in favour of social similarity and viewed the route to liberation in women's equal access to positively valued social positions that have traditionally been the preserve of men. Research on gender inequalities in health grew out of and generally continues within this framework. The other strand has tended to emphasise women's difference from men, has taken the reproductive body as the major site of women's oppression and has viewed the route to liberation in female difference. Research on reproductive health has been associated with this position.

The purpose of this and the following chapter is to raise questions. For example, does this divergent agenda really matter? And, if so, what have been the consequences, both positive and negative, for subsequent research? One response is to say that it has not actually mattered very much given the insights that have been generated. Yet there has been a tendency for the two approaches to talk past each other and, consequently, for a fractured and at times conflicting interpretation of the determinants of women's experience of health and illness to arise. Consequently, it is important to appreciate the broad basis of the different positions in order to evaluate the research agendas that they inspire and the conclusions that they reach, not least because they retain their influence to the present day. As a preliminary it should be noted that, writing in general terms, some commentators believe that distinguishing between different approaches can be useful (see Bradley 2007; Tong 2007), while others are of the opinion that this is bound to lead to inaccuracies since it pushes ideas into boxes, and that it is in any case unhelpful since most of today's feminists work across many different 'schools' (see Wise and Stanley 2003). However, I believe that the two approaches outlined here are theoretically intelligible and therefore constitute a meaningful divide in respect of their influence upon research on health. This said, it is certainly not my intention to argue that *all* feminist health research can be located neatly within one or other approach, but rather to suggest that much of it derives from and has tended to incorporate elements of one or other to varying degrees.

The two approaches, outlined in Table 3.1, are associated with the wider schisms of the 'equality-versus-difference' debate that has haunted feminism since at least the early twentieth century. Plainly put:

> are women to be attributed an identity and sociocultural position in terms that makes it possible for them to be conceived as men's equals? Or are women's identities to be conceived in terms entirely different from those associated with and provided by men?
>
> (Grosz 1995: 49–50).

Research on women's health, which took off in the 1970s, encompasses the two approaches. In its concern with male–female 'equality' and 'social gender' rather than 'biological sex', 'equality feminism' cast a wide net over women's lives, and health was only one concern among many. In contrast, it is nigh impossible to separate issues of health from 'difference feminism' of the same period since it effectively developed through a focus on health and the (reproductive) body.

Equality feminism

Equality or liberal feminism is so strong in the popular imagination that it is often assumed by feminists and non-feminists alike to be *the* feminist approach. As Zillah Eisenstein explains, this is not surprising 'because the state has come to accept this expression of feminism as the least threatening form and, therefore, has given the liberal part of the [women's] movement the most publicity and public recognition' (1981: 177). It is neatly summed up in the words of Betty Friedan: 'to want equality, a voice in the

Table 3.1 Two approaches to women's health

	Equality	*Difference*
Underlying premise	Parity with men	Equal, but different
Operation of patriarchy	Primarily through the social	Primarily through the biological
Way forward	Women's access to valued social spheres	Women's control of the body
Primary research focus	Health status (morbidity and mortality)	Reproductive health

mainstream, to be part of the action of the system: that is what the women's movement is about' (1976: 232; see also Friedan 1981; 1993). The aim, therefore, is not for women to 'take power' but to be included in it on equal terms.

This vision has stood the test of time very well, as witnessed in the new wave of feminist writing that emerged in the 1990s. For example, advancing what she believes to be the radicalism of Friedan's position (Dearey 2006), Naomi Wolf has urged women to regard feminism as a humanist movement in which men should be thought of not as enemies but as partners in a fight for equality where activism is 'a journey to a social contract that includes men and women fairly' (Wolf 1994: 187). The development from around the mid-1990s of the argument that 'men have gender too' has fuelled a high profile 'men's health' lobby that maintains that although they may not be the same, women and men both face disadvantages in society with equally serious consequences for their health (see, for example, Tsuchiya and Williams 2004; White and Cash 2004). In the terms of gender equality politics, this can be thought of as including men in a domain that was once female-defined and therefore as a natural extension of the agenda set in train by equality feminism. 'Gender sensitive' health policy, which is high on the international policy agenda at present (Doyal 2003; UNESCO (United Nations Educational, Scientific and Cultural Organisation) 2003; WHO (World Health Organisation) 2001), is premised on the assumption that making the gender-related experience of both males and females visible 'holds the greatest potential for improving the health of both women and men', that is, for achieving gender equity (Khoury and Weisman 2002: 61). However, it might also be interpreted as an attempt to turn (or return) gender-as-conflict between men and women into gender-as-consensus, that is, into something that, in rather multifarious ways, matters equally for everyone, and thereby as muting feminist agendas.

Although equality feminists recognise that biological specificities exist, the argument is that they should not be allowed to make a difference to life experience. As Elizabeth Grosz explains, there is an assumption that men and women each have 'an analogous biological or natural potential that is unequally developed because the social roles imposed on the two sexes are not equivalent' (1995: 51). Basically, women are as able as men to do what men do, and attention is focused on 'choice and equality of opportunity within existing social relations' (Weedon 1999: 15). It is not surprising, therefore, that women's social roles, and particularly 'dual' or 'multiple' roles, became a major focus of research on gender and health status.

Research on health status

The origins of research on 'gender and health status' were broad based rather than simply feminist inspired. This is what we would expect, given that, as discussed in Chapter 2, the approach to theory building within sociology and the social sciences generally at the time was to include women in, rather than to offer a radical challenge to, existing approaches. Although, for the reasons discussed later in the chapter, much of this early research now seems limited, it was truly groundbreaking at the time and recognised as such by those involved. In fact, the spadework of early equality feminist-inspired research laid a foundation so solid that it remained largely intact and unquestioned until around the mid-1990s.

The observation underlying most research was that, although women in the West were living longer than men – and, indeed, had done so since around the late 1880s – they were sicker (or appeared to be sicker) throughout their lives. From our early twenty-first century vantage point, the early- to mid-1970s appear to have marked a historical peak in the male/female difference in longevity in many western countries that was to be followed by a gradual narrowing (for further discussion, see Chapter 6). But at the time, the gap was felt to be widening in women's favour, a finding that, at least on the surface, seemed at odds with their apparently higher levels of ill health – surely morbidity and mortality are strongly related? The aphorism 'women get sicker but men die quicker' (Nathanson 1977) took a firm and enduring grip on the research agenda. In their attempts to address this apparent anomaly, and also to explore the reasons for differences in health between women, feminists and fellow-travellers sought to do two things: first, to demonstrate that social factors are at least as important – maybe even more important – than biological factors; and, second, to explore the nature of the mechanisms linking social factors with health.

Biology was not cut out of debate entirely; indeed, from the early days researchers lamented the gulf between the 'biological and social camps' of researchers, as Ethel Roskies put it back in the late 1970s (1978: 139; see also Nathanson 1977). It was more a case of arguing that 'inherent' male or female biological advantage/disadvantage could be overridden by social and cultural factors. The abiding intent was to show, largely through quantitative survey research, that social factors really do matter and therefore that any female disadvantage is not 'innate' and fixed but socially created and so changeable. Thus, making an early statement on the 'men die quicker' side of the equation, Ingrid Waldron advised that the role of 'genetic factors' is not as strong as once believed. She suggested that most major causes of death have clear 'behavioural components' linked to the 'masculine role' according to the following 'very rough' proportions: one-third of the male excess may be due to men's higher cigarette smoking (with the major contribution coming from increased risk of coronary heart disease (CHD), lung cancer and emphysema); one-sixth from the greater prevalence of aggressive, competitive, 'coronary prone behaviour' ('Type A' behaviour) among men (itself linked to CHD); one-twelfth from men's higher alcohol consumption (linked to accidents and liver cirrhosis); and one-twentieth being due to the physical hazards that men disproportionately face at work

(Waldron 1976: 357; see also Waldron 1983a, 1983b).[1] Lois Verbrugge also assessed biology's relative contribution, placing it fourth in rank behind: 'risks acquired from roles, stress, life styles, and long-term preventative practices'; psychosocial factors (defined as the possibility that women may report ill health more willingly than men); and prior health care (the tentative suggestion that women's greater contact with health services in earlier life may have a long-term protective effect) (1985: 173).

The apparent anomaly of women's higher morbidity and men's higher age-specific mortality was settled at the time by looking at differences in causes of death and the kinds of illnesses that men and women suffered from. The general conclusion, which tends still to be endorsed today, was that while men suffer from more *serious* illnesses that cause early death, women live on (often into older age) with an excess of chronic, but not necessarily life-threatening illness. Thus Lois Verbrugge summarised the situation as follows:

> Women's days and years are more filled with discomfort and illness restrictions, but contain less threat of life ending from illness. The answer to the question, 'which sex is sicker?' thus varies depending on the timeframe (short versus long run) and the type of health problem (acute versus chronic, fatal versus nonfatal). One sex – women – is indeed sicker in the short run, and the other – men – in the long and ultimate run . . .
>
> (Verbrugge 1988: 139)

However, this did nothing to resolve the knotty question of *how exactly* social factors – if they were important – were influencing health. Early debate focused on the question of whether women's higher morbidity was 'real' – that is, rooted in their material circumstances and/or behaviour – or 'artefactual'; a product of the way that they reported their state of health. Or, to put it another way, do social roles actually make women more ill or just make them appear as if they are more ill? In an agenda-setting paper, Constance Nathanson (1975) outlined three possible reasons for women's higher morbidity: they may *report more illness* in the sense that health is a masculine ethic and it is culturally more acceptable for women to speak about ill health (similar to Verbrugge's 'psychosocial factors', referred to above); the 'sick role' may be more *compatible with women's responsibilities*, in that their 'roles' are purportedly less demanding and they have more time to be sick; they may have more illness due to the *stress of their social roles*. She concluded that the third explanation was the most likely, stating that it is not just that women 'are held to a different, less "adult" standard of health than are men' and/or that they are more willing to express ill health, or have more time to be ill, but that their roles really do seem to make them ill (ibid.: 59). Continuing this line of argument, Walter Gove and Michael Hughes found little empirical support for the artefact explanation and concluded that it is women's 'role obligations', particularly nurturant role demands, which interfere with their ability to care for themselves properly, which lead to higher morbidity. Gove and Hughes and others sought to demonstrate this empirically by showing that, when you control statistically for women's and men's 'role differences', 'sex differences in morbidity largely disappear' (Gove and Hughes 1979: 132). It remains popular for researchers to ask whether there would be any difference in the health status of men and women if they were to occupy similar social positions (see, for example, Bartley 2004; Emslie *et al.* 1999).

Research flourished from these landmark debates as studies sought not only to tease out the reasons why 'women get sicker but men die quicker' but also to consider why some women are sicker than others. Research engaged with the concerns of the time over 'women's place', and questions were posed. For example, if women went out to work, what would it do, not only to their children – would their education suffer, for example? – but also to their own health? Would it all be just too much for them? The answer was a fairly resounding 'no'. It should be recalled that the theme of 'women, work and marriage' had been brought to the heart of wider feminism by this time (as discussed in Chapter 2). Kate Millett, for example, had declared the family to be patriarchy's chief institution, 'both a mirror of and a connection with the larger society; a patriarchal unit within a patriarchal whole' (1970: 33). Diana Leonard Barker and Sheila Allen had argued that the traditional sociological division between research on the home and research on paid work needed to be re-cast to consider the systematic interrelationships between them. A swathe of hitherto unexplored questions were being posed such as:

> what are the differences between work in the home, the unpaid servicing of family members, which has not as yet been prominent among the concerns of the sociologists of work, and that outside the domestic group which is paid and has been studied for many decades by industrial sociology? If we seek social change, at what points in the structure can we most effectively 'insert a lever'?
>
> (Barker and Allen 1976: 3)

Sheila Rowbotham wrote about the 'neurosis of nothingness' that results from the women's work in the home. Under the heading 'A woman's work is never done', she argued in her book *Woman's Consciousness in a Man's World* that although there are strong links between economic deprivation and health, 'there are illnesses which have nothing to do with poverty, which come simply from being housebound and being a woman in capitalist society' (1973: 76).

Following the contention that the route to positive health lies in access to hitherto male-defined spheres, researchers in the health field thus began to demonstrate that it was 'housewives' who suffered most from ill-health, not women in paid employment (and that this could not be accounted for by the effect of more healthy women working, or what is known as 'health selection'). Nathanson (1975) and others pointed out that although paid work can be a source of stress, it can also be health protective because it is 'socially integrating' and benefits self-esteem through feelings of accomplishment. Housework, by contrast, is monotonous, arduous and 'never done', stressful and socially isolating (Oakley 1974a, 1974b; Rowbotham 1973). Drawing on the wider theory of social support and health, researchers also began to explore the relationship between marriage and health. Walter Gove (1972), for example, found that the 'interpersonal ties' of marriage were good for the health of both men and women (unmarried people seemed to fare much worse), but that the benefits were greater for men than for women, a finding that, broadly speaking, has been replicated subsequently (Nathanson 1977; Bird and Rieker 2008). This echoes the centuries-old concern of writers such as Mary Astell and Charlotte Perkins Gilman, discussed in Chapter 1, that marriage reflects women's dependence and, more often than not, is the root of their physical and mental deterioration.

As research developed into the 1980s and beyond, a range of other variables – such as age and social class, parenthood, the type of work that people do, whether work is full or part time, the composition of households, and the 'quality' of relationships – were incorporated into analyses. This has culminated in a wealth of research on the question of whether so-called 'multiple roles' are a source of strain resulting in overload and felt conflict (and therefore negative for health, or for aspects of health) or whether what has variously been called role enhancement, role expansion or role accumulation is beneficial. The general conclusion of early research was that multiple roles were beneficial; entering the 'male world' even while retaining one's traditional commitments in the home did not seem to cause major harm, at least when the conditions of each were favourable (Verbrugge 1983), a finding that generally still holds unless demands and time pressures tip over into severe 'role overload' (Bird and Rieker 2008; Härenstam *et al.* 2001; McMunn *et al.* 2006). Recently researchers have explored the juggling that women engage in as they negotiate (as far as this is possible) what is conceptualised as 'work–life balance', 'work–life conflict' or negative 'spillover', addressing the balance of harmful and beneficial effects of multiple roles on health in relation to specific role combinations, role characteristics and conditions of work (see, for example, Bird and Rieker 2008; Doyal 1995; McMunn *et al.* 2006; Waldron *et al.* 1998). Research has also developed beyond the fairly basic measures of 'role occupancy' that characterised early studies to take account of the quality and meaning, or lived experience, of domestic and paid work using concepts such as 'role involvement' and 'role commitment' (see, for example, Nazroo *et al.* 1998).

A critical reflection

The conceptual power of this strand of research is evident in its lasting influence. Indeed it was not subject to any significant critique until around the mid-1990s, by which time there was an emerging sense that it was losing direction, becoming confusing and inconsistent, and even that it had reached a log-jam or conceptual impasse (Kandrack *et al.* 1991). There are two major problems that researchers are slowly beginning to address. First, although a distinction between the social (gender) and the biological (sex) may be a necessary first step in challenging the patriarchal conflation of women with their biology, construing the relationship as more or less arbitrary is a problematic basis on which to rest an analysis of health. A second related problem is the reduction of the social relations of gender and women's health to something that happens to social roles conceived as the properties of individuals. Each of these problems will now be briefly discussed.

Separating the social and the biological

While feminists were wrapped up with the social, biologists and medical scientists were hot on their heels An exemplar of this is the growing backlash specialism of 'gender specific medicine' (see Legato 2003a, 2003b), which, despite the name and despite the lip service given to social factors, is overwhelmingly concerned with explaining differences in the health of men and women in biological terms (Grace 2007; see also the discussion in Chapter 5). It is an illustration of what feminist biologist Anne Fausto-Sterling dubs the 'spreading oil spill of sex' (Fausto-Sterling 2005: 1495) and a grave warning sign that it is not possible to counter the patriarchal conflation of women with their biology by proposing that biology does not really matter. Instead, biology needs to be brought back into the feminist fold.

As Nancy Krieger explains:

> although lucid analyses have been written on why it is important to distinguish between 'gender' and 'sex', epidemiological and other health research has been hampered by a lack of clear conceptual models for considering *both*, simultaneously, to determine their relevance – or not – to the outcome(s) being researched.
>
> (2003: 653, emphasis in original)

The line of argument here, and more widely, is not that we should abandon the sex (biology)/gender (social) distinction. Indeed, by and large the line of reasoning is that if we conflate the two, this 'reinforces erroneous beliefs that experiences of gender are about biology' (Krieger and Zierler 1995: 252). Rather, the contention is that we need to know how sex (biology) and social (gender) each operate in relation to specific disease processes or overall health status in order that we might then explore how they might interact (see also Doyal 2003; Kandrack *et al.* 1991; Payne 2006). But, as commentators appreciate, it is one thing to state this and quite another to develop an analytic framework to actually study this process. As feminist biologist Lynda Birke points out, writing in more general terms, a good part of the problem is that the biological has 'become a kind of ragbag into which a highly heterogenous and eclectic mix of stuff can be thrown' (1999: 31). Health researchers generally agree that relevant biological differences are likely to go beyond the reproductive to include hormonal, genetic and metabolic influences (Bird and Rieker 2008; Doyal 2001; Krieger 2003; Payne 2006), but the decisive question of what *it is* about biology that matters remains largely unanswered at the present time.

Two useful attempts to develop integrative frameworks are Nancy Krieger's 'ecosocial perspective' and Chloe Bird and Patricia Rieker's 'constrained choices' approach. Krieger's 'ecosocial perspective' is a highly ambitious attempt to map conceptually the myriad interlocking social and biological processes that work at every level – cell, organ, organism; individual, family, community; population, society, ecosystem – to produce embodied health inequalities, not only in relation to women and men, as is our concern here, but more generally to include social class, ethnicity and other factors (Krieger 2001). Referring specifically to sex and gender, she presents twelve case studies to explore the circumstances in which 'gender relations and sex-linked biology are singly, neither, or both relevant to independent or synergistic determinants' of health outcomes (Krieger 2003: 653). These are diverse and very specific, and include, for example, the prevalence of contact lens microbial keratitis (inflammation of the cornea), age of HIV infection among women compared to heterosexual men, and health outcomes due to ubiquitous exposure to cooking oil contaminated by polychlorinated biphenyls (PCB) ('Yusho' disease). Bird and Rieker's (2008) 'constrained choices' model foregrounds the 'personal choices' that men and women make in relation to their health as they are shaped by wider social policies and the communities within which they live. They emphasise that the relationship between the levels of policy, community, and individual health choices is highly complex and that, 'few if any researchers have attempted to marshall the data needed either to specify those connections or clarify the role of biological processes in this dynamic' (ibid.: 183).

These integrative frameworks are useful for their attempts to draw the relationship between the biological and the social into a wider theory of the production of health. However, as the above quotation from Bird and Rieker makes patently clear, in practical terms research insights are really quite limited. Studies appear to have been most successful when they have addressed specific health conditions in relation to specific life circum-stances. A well-worked example is Sarah Payne's (2004) analysis of existing published research on irritable bowel syndrome (IBS). IBS, which affects between 20 and 40 per cent of the UK population, has a much higher incidence among women. Given that women are more susceptible during particular phases of the reproductive cycle, biological risks are thought to be related to hormonal factors. IBS is also associated with stress and anxiety in both male and female sufferers, but women with the condition are more likely to report feelings of severe anxiety, depression, tiredness, crying and sleep loss (which in themselves are more common in women). Payne therefore concludes that 'there may be common causes of stress, poor health, and IBS that reflect gender relations' (ibid.: 22); that is, the higher incidence of IBS among women may result from a combination of biological factors and the stressful conditions of their lives. Although, of themselves, analyses of this kind are very useful, they are at some remove from the wider integrative frameworks discussed above. At present, then, there is something of a gulf between conceptual models and empirical analysis, which leaves us ill-equipped to understand the role of the biological (sex) and the social (gender), and their possible interaction, in relation to wider patterns of morbidity.

Reductivism

The second problem afflicting much research on 'gender and health status' is its highly reductivist character. Health and illness are framed as something that 'happens' to social roles defined as properties of individuals rather than, as is more appropriate, something that is experienced by embodied individuals in particular social milieu. The concepts of 'social roles' and 'gender roles' are still used in a multiplicity of ways, almost to the point that they seem to refer loosely to anything that has social, rather than bio-logical, connotations. Variables such as women's work, marital and parental status, household structure and social class, for example, are variously defined as components of social roles, social positions or social statuses, which, in their turn, are rarely defined or distinguished. As Jennie Popay and Keleigh Groves discuss, much past and current research 'seeks to represent and explore patterns of morbidity between women and men using measures which in large part have no theoretical basis and which can be and are changed in important ways at the "whim" of the researcher' (2000: 74).

Given that the social role framework was already being significantly contested within wider sociology by the late 1970s, it may seem surprising that it has remained so prominent in 'gender and health' research for so long. As John Hood-Williams put it, although not referring to health, 'the familiar functionalist concepts of "role" and "socialisation" . . . had a new feminist vibrancy breathed into them at a time in the history of sociology when many thought they had permanently expired' (1996: 5). However, the relative durability of these concepts within sociological research on health specifically is perhaps easier to understand. Talcott Parsons' concept of the 'sick role' was a powerful influence upon the newly establishing medical sociology of the 1960s and 1970s (Parsons 1950). It was part of the wider endeavour to capture the social as the domain of sociology in distinction to the biological, which belonged to the discipline of medicine. This, alongside its conceptual fit with equality or liberal feminism, may explain why it has taken longer for the social role framework to be questioned in research on gender and health than in other areas.

In early studies in particular, social roles had a heavily scripted character, so much so that researchers often made assumptions of male/female difference from the outset – what would matter for women, what for men – which, rather ironically, meant that they often replicated the very bi-polar social script (discussed in Chapter 2) that they were aiming to challenge. To be sure, researchers are now increasingly alert to these kinds of problems, and, as a consequence, studies are becoming more nuanced and sensitive to the complexities of women's and men's lives. As Sally Macintyre and colleagues report, the supposition that women have a greater propensity to report more ill health than men (at a given level of symptomatology) has had a long shelf life, so much so that it has taken on the character of an urban folk tale (Macintyre *et al.* 1999: 91). A growing number of researchers are now voicing the opinion that too many taken-for-granted assumptions, such as the universality of women's higher (and men's lower) morbidity, have been allowed to continue unchecked (see, for example, Annandale 1998a, 1998b; Gorman and Ghazal Read 2006; Lahelma *et al.* 2001; McDonough and Walters 2001; Macintyre *et al.* 1996; Payne 2006). But despite the awakening of researchers to the need to appreciate the diversity of women's experience, searches for ways to explore the interaction of the biological and the social and endeavours to take account of social change in women's lives, there is still a general reluctance among researchers to theorise how the social relations of gender in society actually operate to influence health. All too often research still stops at the point of stating that things are more complex than hitherto was assumed, without analysing what it is that is happening in society and the social relations of gender to account for this.

When research focuses only on a cluster of proximate causes, gender and health lose their social structural moorings. For example, a recent review of research published between 1950 and 2000 on 'women, work and well-being' by Petra Klumb and Thomas Lampert (2004) confirms that the effects of employment on women's health and well-being are either positive or neutral, rather than negative. They rightly conclude that the usefulness of these studies is limited due to their lack of theoretical underpinning. But by this they appear simply to mean a lack of clear, testable hypotheses and the relative failure to attend to the psychosocial processes that are likely to mediate between employment and health, such as a personal sense of mastery or competence and social affirmation through social interaction. They conspicuously fail to make any reference to wider social relations of gender.

This neglect is intrinsic to the paradigm of research on social inequalities in health of which gender and health status research is part. As Janet Shim explains, this body of research has a very strong tendency to distil the effects of social and relational ideologies, structures and practices organised around 'race', gender and social class:

> into characteristics of discrete and self-contained individuals. Disciplinary paradigms and practices effectively deny that historical changes in social policies, ideologies and prevailing meanings of difference 'get under the skin' and fundamentally affect well-being. Epidemiology thereby renders invisible the very social relations of power structuring material and psychic conditions and life chances that contribute to the stratification of health.
>
> (Shim 2002: 134)

Crucially, without these structural moorings we are left with findings – similarities and differences on various measures of health – for which we have no real explanation. Gayle Rubin's (1975) stress on the *systemic* character of the sex/gender distinction, mentioned in Chapter 2, was an early warning signal that our attention should be directed as much towards the underlying processes – such as the particular form that patriarchy takes in time and place – which make certain kinds of knowledge possible, as to the analysis of the content of particular 'social roles' or aggregate measures. As Judith Stacey and Barrie Thorne put it back in the mid-1980s, the notion of social roles is depoliticising since 'they strip experience from its historical and political context and neglect questions of power and context' (1985: 307). Gender is at heart a relational concept that connotes structural relations of inequality, which do not simply imply difference but also hierarchies of power (Busfield 1996). Therefore we need to forge 'new methodological approaches to show how *gender oppression* – as opposed to an uncomplicated epidemiological variable of *gender* – shapes women's health outcomes and well-being' (Inhorn and Whittle 2001: 564, emphasis in original). This necessitates connecting women's lived experiences of health and illness and 'the various forms of oppression that they encounter to larger social, economic and political forces' (ibid.: 564).

Arguably some progress has been made in this regard in recent attempts by quantitative researchers to incorporate measures of the macro 'gendered context' into research. An early and highly influential example of this is research by Ichiro Kawachi and colleagues in the US, which modelled women's health status as an 'ecological characteristic' (Kawachi *et al.* 1999: 21). Composite indicators of women's political participation, economic autonomy, employment and earnings, and reproductive rights at the state level were assessed for their ability to explain total mortality rates, cause-specific mortality, and the average days of activity limitation that women had experienced in the previous month. They found that the measures of women's health were 'strikingly correlated' with each of these state-level measures, leading them to conclude that 'women experience higher mortality and morbidity in states where they have lower levels of political participation and economic autonomy' (ibid.: 21). As they appreciate, modelling women's health status as an ecological characteristic risks what is known as the ecological fallacy, that is, assuming that the health of individual women can be explained by aggregate statistics for states as a whole. Subsequently, researchers have employed the statistical technique of multi-level modelling to distinguish between what are known as *contextual*, or macro-level, and *compositional*, or individual level, effects upon health. For example, Ying-Yeh Chen and colleagues (2005) modelled the relationship between women's status and autonomy at the state level and depressive symptoms, also taking account of the characteristics of individual women who lived in (or composed) the state, such as age, ethnicity, income, education and employment status, that is, compositional effects. They found that although women with lower socio-economic status and ethnic minorities had more symptoms, *all* women benefited from living in US states that were more equal, that is, the contextual effects of the macro gender context were important influences.

Nancy Moss concludes that 'contextualizing studies in historical and geopolitical frameworks is a next big step' in attempts to develop an integrated framework for research on women's health status (2002: 659). However, so far, research on contextual effects that explicitly builds measures of macro-level 'gender inequality' into analysis has been limited. And, as many researchers working within this framework are aware, the conceptual gap between macro-level variables such as political participation and levels of women's employment and women's individual-level characteristics needs to be filled in with variables that tap into features of the local community or neighbourhood, since the pathways between health and features such as immediate physical environment, access to amenities such as shops, levels of crime and so on may be different for men and women. For example, researching urban neighbourhoods in Stockholm, Sweden, Kristina Sundquist and colleagues (2006) found that in neighbourhoods with the highest levels of violent crime, the odds of developing coronary heart disease were 1.77 for women and only 1.39 for men. In neighbourhoods with the highest unemployment rates, the corresponding odds ratios were 2.05 and 1.50. This suggests that men and women may experience the gendered context differently (Bird and Rieker 2008), something that may be better captured by qualitative research that attends to how people relate to places (Popay and Groves 2000). Moreover, as Bird and Rieker (2008) discuss, it is possible that men and women may have different physiological responses to stressors which lead them to adopt different 'coping styles', which then affect health behaviours such as cigarette smoking, exercise, alcohol consumption and diet. However, as they go on to explain, much more research is needed to examine and elucidate the role of biology in this process, which has been conspicuously absent in this body of research to date.

Conclusion

The chapter began by outlining two different approaches to women's health that grew out of feminists' early use of the sex/gender distinction. For 'equality feminists', rather than being a straightforward product of their biology, women's heath is socially constructed through their occupancy of gender-specific statuses and the enactment of gender-related social roles. From this perspective the biological tends to collapse into the social, thereby muting its explanatory potential. This alone is problematic, but there are also difficulties with the conceptualisation of the social itself. While the wider social, economic and political forces that structure women's oppressions are clearly the point of reference, there is a marked propensity for women's lived experience to be distilled into proximate causes. Explanatory power then becomes invested in individuals as carriers of certain social roles and statuses. The second approach to research on gender and health outlined in Table 3.1 would appear to have a ready answer to how the social relations of gender operate: patriarchy is the root of oppression for all women and the biological body is the primary site of women's oppression. Moreover, it seems to offer 'a visceral, tangible sense of alternatives' (Di Stefano 1990: 71), which lies in casting off male–medical explications of women's biological inferiority in favour of positive, woman-centred definitions of health and the body. As will be discussed in Chapter 4, conceptualised as the pre-eminent – and often vexed – juncture around which women's lives pivot, reproduction became for many the rallying point for an analysis of women's oppression under patriarchy.

4　Women and reproduction

Introduction

I have argued that the conceptual coffers of the sex (biology)/gender (social) distinction were a treasure trove for research on women's health. The distinction generated two lines of argument with two rather different research foci. While, as discussed in Chapter 3, equality feminism challenged the patriarchal equation of (biological) sex and (social) gender by drawing attention to the *social* nature of women's oppression, difference or radical feminism emphasised the oppression of women through the body, or *biology*. Rather than claiming that women's biology is inferior (patriarchy) or not particularly salient (equality feminism), from the perspective of 'difference' or radical feminism, revaluing women's biological capacity is essential to their well-being.

I begin this chapter by sketching how a growing interest in maternity as a transition point in women's lives drew reproduction and childbirth to the heart of the sociological endeavour, not simply as a resource to explore wider sociological concerns, as hitherto had been the case (see Chapter 2), but as a vital ingredient for the analysis of women's oppression in its own right. Although most commentators appreciate that it is meaningless to think in terms of 'pure biology' in the sense of a 'natural' female body, traces of essentialism nonetheless run through much feminist research on birth. This is evident in the prevailing oppositional discourse, which evokes a natural reproductive body in order to counter the distortions of patriarchal medicine. Two models of childbirth – one natural and female controlled, the other unnatural and male-controlled – continue to animate the research agenda. The consequence is a tendency to set research and critical commentary within a framework of difference.

Reproduction, the family and the social relations of gender

As we began to see in Chapter 3, during the 1970s a new generation of female sociologists and others struggled to bring health and gender to the heart of sociological analysis. The objective was not only to illuminate women's health concerns – although that was achievement enough – but to undertake the more fundamental task of arguing that the association between gender and health was actually key to the wider social relations of gender. For the reasons outlined in Chapter 2, this was a long hard journey, and one that is still being taken today. Feminist academics, sociologists included, were beginning to appreciate, as Robin Saltonstall (1993) was later to elaborate, that it was not simply that gender could help us to understand health but that health could help us to understand gender. This prompted those who might not have been interested in health per se to appreciate its potential. The central place of reproduction in this enterprise is not surprising since it came to be seen as the pre-eminent – and often vexed – juncture around which women's lives pivoted. As Ann Oakley put it, 'a repossession of female control over reproductive care is a basic prerequisite for all freedoms' (1976: 58).

Alice Rossi (1968) pointed out that up to this point research on maternity and parenting had been directed almost exclusively towards what the child needs from the mother, while women's own experience, especially privations such as reduced involvement in non-family activities, had been totally neglected. Concerns such as Rossi's need to be situated in relation to the bi-polar social script discussed in Chapter 2. Although women's employment and employment rights were being actively campaigned for, wider social attitudes were slow to move away from traditional expectations of women's domestic and maternal roles in the home. Tradition and change sat uneasily side by side, prompting all kinds of anxiety. Researchers began to argue that maternity was taking the place of marriage as the major transition point in women's lives. Rossi explained that pregnancy and parenthood disrupted the expectations of young women who had been 'reared with highly diversified interests and social expectations concerning adult life' and that this was leading 'to a depressed sense of self worth' (1968: 27, 34). Similarly, Ann Oakley (1975) argued that the main factor marking the difference between the lives of twenty-five year olds during the early to mid-1970s and those of their grandmothers' generation was not, as was conventionally believed, changes in education and employment but those in reproduction. Life had become much more complicated, since women's identity was now doubly defined in terms of paid employment and being a housewife. Specifically, the fact that they no longer simply 'gave up' their work for marriage in the manner of their grandmothers had, made 'the birth of a first child an unequalled crisis for women' (ibid.: 640). Interestingly, Oakley tied this to the preoccupation – clearly popular even in the mid-1970s – of whether 'women are becoming more like men and men more like women', arguing that the unknown effects of the medicalisation of childbirth, such as mental and emotional problems, needed to be taken seriously as factors that could stall the narrowing gap between the social behaviour of men and women (ibid.: 639).

But in taking up these issues researchers faced a problem: there simply was no useful body of research to draw upon. It can be difficult looking back after the subsequent outpouring of research to appreciate that, back in the mid-1970s, there was a dearth of academic research on the experience of childbirth. As Oakley put it, there was 'no study of childbirth from the woman's point of view', only personal accounts and impressions (1976: 21; see also Rapp 2001). The lack of knowledge about 'normal' birth in different cultures was hardly surprising given that, up to that point, most research had been carried out by male anthropologists who did not have access to women's spheres (Rich 1977). Within sociology, the prevailing ethos was to approach reproduction through marriage and the family, topics that, as discussed in Chapter 2, were highly influenced by structural functionalism. Maternity was construed as a marital affair, of interest only insofar as it was a woman's passport to proper femininity and the affirmation of her normative role within the family as the emotional carer of children. Thus, as Oakley put it, the failure of sociologists to 'detach themselves from prevailing cultural norms' distanced women from their own experiences (1980: 78). For example, in *Family and Kinship in Modern Britain*, Christopher Turner (1969) simply took it for granted, and thereby tacitly accepted, that childbearing and childrearing would curtail the mother's activities outside the home. The related failure by sociologists to problematise notions such as maternal instinct and its corollaries, such as the belief that childbearing is woman's highest, yet most basic, function, meant that 'normal' reproduction was taken for granted as part of the natural order (Macintyre 1978). When reproduction *was* considered, it was the 'problematic' such as abortion, illegitimacy and 'single mothers' that drew attention. As Sally Macintyre (1978) discussed, 'single mothers' could not fail to be anything other than a disturbance to the social order when it was assumed that single women do not want to be (and should not be) pregnant.

The yoking of reproductive activities to marriage and the family had also deflected attention away from a critical analysis of the profession of obstetrics and gynaecology (Oakley 1980), which, to the extent that it was contemplated at all, was positioned as a neutral player as researchers focused on matters such as women's lack of compliance with medical regimens and missed attendance at antenatal clinics. Medicine's role was to police normal pregnancy and birth and to sort things out when they 'went wrong', such as when pregnancy and birth occurred outside of marriage. In sum, medico-centrism and the normative assumptions inherent in prevailing research on the family resulted in an embryonic sociology of reproduction ensnared in the assumption that woman's normative maternal role flowed from her biology. The feminist challenge rested upon making clear that givens, such as 'maternal instinct', were socially constructed. This challenged the yoking of reproduction to marriage and, to paraphrase Sally Macintyre (1978), the assumption that people have babies because they are married, or marry in order to have babies; that people have babies because they have had sex, or that they have sex in order to produce babies.

Medicine quite quickly became politically laden within sociology as its purported neutrality was questioned. For example, Macintyre's (1977) research revealed that assumptions on the part of doctors that marriage and motherhood are women's natural role in life had a marked impact on the care that they received when single and pregnant. She showed that the assumptions of British general practitioners that childbirth was only acceptable within marriage highly coloured their response to patients. Those who intended to get married were treated 'as-if-married' and encouraged not to terminate their pregnancies. Those who did not intend to get married were categorised either as 'good' girls, who were typically young, had used birth control and were known by them, or as 'bad' girls, who were judged to be promiscuous, had a past history of vaginal infections and did not use birth control. Whereas good girls who could give a valid reason for why they could not get married were usually referred for an abortion, bad girls were typically punished and not referred. Kristen Luker's (1975) study of a Californian abortion clinic also drew attention to the association between the acceptability of contraceptive 'risk taking' and marital status. Although abortion was legally permitted on certain grounds, the total number of women seeking terminations on grounds of rape, incest or threat to physical health was less than 5 per cent. Consequently, most presented 'a threat to mental health' as their reason for abortion, and this required a psychiatric examination. Even though, more often than not, this was a ritual step in 'earning' an abortion, it still involved a process of labelling based on marital status. Luker found that married women were far more likely to have their pregnancy put down to contraceptive failure and to be diagnosed as having 'transitional situational disturbances' than as having personality disorders or depressive neuroses. The latter diagnoses were more likely to be reserved for widowed, divorced or separated women – women who should have 'known better' than to get pregnant. Luker concludes that this difference probably occurred 'because a woman's social category triggers certain assumptions in the minds of those who put labels on her as she goes through an abortion clinic' (ibid.: 39).

Since it was now seen as foundational to women's life chances, reproduction became the centrepiece of feminist endeavours to challenge the existing androcentric sociology. The sex (biology)/gender (social) distinction was drawn upon to counter the normative assumptions – held within medicine and more widely – that women's biology is their destiny. This meant showing that the female biological body is invested with problematic social ideologies that have been imported into medical and social science. Researchers turned to topics such as the dynamics of interaction between the male dominated medical profession and female patients and their consequences for quality of care (e.g. Doyal 1979; Fisher 1984; Fisher and Groce 1985; Scully and Bart 1973; Shapiro *et al.* 1983; Wallen *et al.*

1979). But, for some, the problem ran a lot deeper than questioning particular biological ascriptions; female biology itself needed to be radically revalued.

Pure difference?

Frequently maligned and often wilfully misunderstood (Morgan 1996; Stanley and Wise 1993), radical or 'difference feminism' is not only the feminism that the media loves to hate (Zalewski 2000) but also the feminism that other feminists often disparage. Radical feminism has the character of a dancing light – iridescent and full of colour but difficult to pin down. As Marysia Zalewski remarks:

> [it is] susceptible to being presented in ways that make it easy to dismiss it as outdated and over the top. There has been a tendency, amongst feminists and non-feminists alike, to look back to the early texts and search out the most outrageous and dogmatic statements and use them as evidence of radical feminism's contemporary uselessness.
>
> (Zalewski 2000: 14–15)

It is my contention that, even though the influence of the radical feminist vision of the 1970s and early 1980s has diminished with time, its influence lives on in research on reproduction and childbirth. It is therefore important to capture its underlying premises. One way of trying to avoid the kind of distortion that Zalewski refers to is to use its proponents' own words. Thus Elaine Morgan makes clear what radical feminism is *not*. It is not socialist or Marxist feminism, since from that perspective patriarchy is simply the by-product of capitalism and women will be free when capitalism has been superseded. It is not liberal or 'equality feminism' since, as she puts it, this kind of feminism plays by patriarchy's own rules. By assuming that 'imitating establishment men' is good for women, 'equality feminism' settles for a 'piece of the pie as currently and poisonously baked' (Morgan 1996: 5). Thus the very rights to which equality feminists aspire are not simply male-defined, but defined *against* women (a point also made by critics of equality feminism from other theoretical perspectives; see, for example, Gatens 1983; Jaggar 1983; Vogel 1995). Women have not simply been excluded from the rational (male) world of reason; rationality itself has been defined against them by denying the specificity of the female body. Treating women as equal to men will not always produce fair results for women; the special needs of pregnant women in employment, for example, could be denied.

Robyn Rowland and Renate Klein concretise radical feminism in two tenets: first and foremost, 'women as a social group are oppressed by men as a social group and ... this oppression is the *primary* oppression for women'; second, it is woman-centred, created 'by women for women' (1996: 11, emphasis in original). Although patriarchy differs in form across time and place, it is universal in its impact: all women are oppressed, though in different ways and to different extents. Women therefore always exist as a social caste or class. This means that, although differences between them such as those based on 'race', age and social class matter, more often than not, they are superseded by their interests qua women. In this conceptualisation women's common biological difference to men will always matter. As Rowland and Klein argue, 'internationally, it is a woman's body which is the currency of patriarchy' (ibid.: 17) and the major site of women's oppression, witnessed in the worldwide experience of rape, violence, forced pregnancy and sexual slavery (pornography, sex tourism, the international traffic in women).

From this perspective the notion of androgyny – or the mixture of feminine and masculine virtues, or a vision of a world where gender is no longer relevant, espoused by authors such as Judith Lorber, who writes that she would 'like to see the genders unified (degendered) as a way of repairing the world' (Lorber 2005: 5) – is a ploy on the part of men, since all it intends is to eliminate the powerful female presence. In this sense, the summary, 'equal, but different' depicted in Table 3.1 (Chapter 3) does not do justice to this stronger position since, for some, it is not just a matter of appreciating women's 'difference' from men, or even of recognising that, untrammelled by patriarchy, women's physicality is in many ways superior and powerful; it is a matter of rejecting 'difference *from*' and asserting a positive difference outside the patriarchal binary.

Philosopher and theologian Mary Daly (1984) insists that androgyny is men's last-ditch attempt to invite women into the patriarchal plot by appropriating all that is best about women. Patriarchy, she argues, has deprived women of their bona fide passions and substituted 'plastic' or 'potted' versions in their place. Daly's thesis comprises a double move: the transvaluation of patriarchal ascriptions and the revaluing of women's 'true nature'. Her ambition in writing the book *Pure Lust* was to inspire women to release themselves from the pots and plastic moulds blocking their passions. She argues that once patriarchal notions such as 'femininity' are stripped away, women can experience their original (pre-patriarchal) female power. Terms such as 'hag', 'crone' and 'spinster' become the metaphors for women's creation of a new culture beyond patriarchy.

The writing of Mary Daly – and the poetry and prose of others such as Adrienne Rich – has a visceral power that convinces with not only the 'sharp clarity of its substantive position but the sheer force if its literary style – so able to move the heart, and surely almost able to move the world' (Cocks 1988: 30). It evokes an idea of the self as a 'vital, passionate being' (ibid.: 30). This is very apparent in the early writing of Susan Griffin who, in the preface to the book *Woman and Nature*, remarks: 'my prose in this book is like poetry, and like poetry always begins with feeling'

(1978: xv). Her voice in the book is embodied and impassioned. In the place of what she calls patriarchy's 'separations' – of mind and emotion, body and soul – she envisions a different way of seeing through women's deep connection with nature.

By transvaluing the male connection where the female body is a vessel of death – wilful, evil, devouring, even deadly – women gain their new space. Thus Griffin writes:

> Her space *The cosmos* flooded with *The Earth* her vision. The space where her feelings pulled her apart and what was inside her was revealed. And this lit her way. Space where, in her circling motion, she found an opening ... We know ourselves to be made from this earth. We know this earth is made from our bodies. For we see ourselves. And we are nature. We are nature seeing nature. We are nature with a concept of nature. Nature weeping. Nature speaking of nature to nature.
>
> (Griffin 1978: 171, 226)

Here woman's nature and nature in her connection with woman are separate from – and superior to – *man*ufactured culture. Daly (1993) conceptualises feminists as 'outercoursing', moving beyond the imprisoning mental, physical, emotional and spiritual walls of patriarchy (the state of possession) to find their elemental connections with the natural world and each other. In *Pure Lust*, she formulates a new philosophy, a new way of being for women that is in harmony with nature, where the force of reason is 'rooted in instinct, intuition, passion' (1984: 7).

Reproduction and the body politic

It is important to appreciate the distinction between what has been viewed critically by some as the individualising tendencies of early feminist health activism (Bell 1994; Bell and Reverby 2005; Kuhlmann forthcoming), discussed in Chapter 2, and the feminist philosophy outlined above. Susan Griffin, Mary Daly and others approach the female body from the vantage point that it is the *body politic* that matters. Rejecting the distanced and purportedly objective 'masculine' stance, their writing on women and the reproductive body is embodied insofar as it grows from experience. For some, reproduction became a trope for the 'doing' of feminist theory itself. Mary O'Brien, for example, referred to feminists 'labouring to give birth to a new philosophy of birth', which will show that male dominance is much more than economic in form (1981: 17). In turning attention from the social relations of production to the social relations of *re*production, many feminists – sociologists included – saw themselves as engaging critically with Marx's materialist conception of history and with the debate over the relative primacy of social class and gender as organising principles, which was dominant within sociology and the social sciences generally during the 1970s and early 1980s. Although they recognised that social class could divide women, they nonetheless maintained that, above all, women exist as a 'sex class', and this was the principle that drove the theoretical agenda on reproductive health forward. For many it was not so much a matter of jettisoning Marx's dialectical and material conception of history but of turning it to feminism's advantage by extending it to encompass socially reproductive or procreative labour.

However, it can be argued that feminists sympathetic to Marxism did not give reproduction the attention that it deserved during the 1970s and early 1980s. This was the case despite some support for the importance of reproduction in Friedrich Engels' *Origin of the Family, Private Property and the State* (1972 [1844]). Thus Nicky Hart later argued that, following the lead of classical social theory, they had 'abandoned procreation to a pre-social "natural" backwater, accepting that its social relations caused no more than a ripple on the surface of real material life – the production of saleable goods and services' (1996: 27). Although latterly feminists have conceded this neglect, many have remained wary of any latent 'biologism' inherent in the emphasis on women's 'unique' reproductive functions. Juliet Mitchell, for example, emphasises that 'it is important that the difficult question of the social place of motherhood, which is historically variable, does not collapse into the timeless mystique of earth-motherdom' (1996: 50). Given these disputes, it should come as no surprise that reproduction quickly became not only the rallying point for feminist health politics but also a rather bloody theoretical battle ground in its own right.

Firestone and O'Brien

This was thrown into early relief in the 1970s in the contrasting views of Shulamith Firestone and Mary O'Brien. In the subtitle to her book *The Dialectic of Sex,* 'the case for a feminist revolution', Firestone signals that her concern extends way beyond reproduction per se. Reproduction is, in her own words, the driving force of history. But women have been dealt a cruel hand: a biologically based 'sexual imbalance of power' based on their childbearing and childrearing roles (Firestone 1971: 10). Nature has set up oppressive power structures that have been 'reinforced by man' through the cult of romance and the tyranny of the biological family, which yokes women to men (ibid.: 16). Women are a slave class that exists to maintain the species in order to free men for the business of the world. In Firestone's view, there is no more reason to accept this 'biological disadvantage' than there is to accept bourgeois rule. In the same way that workers' liberation necessitates the overthrow of the means of production, women's liberation demands the overthrow of the means of *re*production: the false dichotomy that biology has created between men and women must be swept away. Seizure of the control of reproduction will restore women's ownership of their own bodies to themselves, along with 'feminine control of human fertility, including the new technology and all the social institutions of childbearing' (ibid.: 11). Just as proletarian class action will eventually destroy not only bourgeois private property but the whole notion of private property, feminist action will eliminate not only male privilege but the relevance of the biological (sex) distinction itself. As Firestone puts it, genital differences between human beings would no longer be of cultural or political importance.

In somewhat emotive terms, Firestone writes that feminists now 'have the knowledge to create a paradise on earth anew' (ibid.: 272). The harbinger of this new freedom is reproductive technology. At the time of writing in the late 1960s, Firestone's reference to ectogenesis belonged far more to the realms of fantasy than reality (Wajcman 1991; 2004). She stipulates using every means available to free women from their reproductive tyranny, from artificial contraception to 'more distant solutions based on the potentials of modern embryology', that is, artificial reproduction, the possibilities of which, she felt, were still so frightening that they were seldom discussed seriously (Firestone 1971: 233).What about the so-called joy of childbirth? It is just a myth. Anticipating disapproval from the women's movement and what she called the 'cult of natural childbirth', Firestone insisted that childbirth is barbaric, maintaining that when the blood tie to the mother is broken by technology, the role of childbearing and childrearing can be diffused to society as a whole, 'to men and other children as well as women' (ibid.: 270). Pregnancy, which is 'clumsy, inefficient, and painful would be indulged in, if at all, only as a tongue-in-cheek archaism' (ibid.: 274).

The critical responses to Firestone's thesis are well known: pregnancy and childbirth are not inherently barbaric; it is not biology that has dealt women a cruel hand, but patriarchal control of it. By resorting to technological control of reproduction, women are giving away their ability to give life. *The Dialectic of Sex* certainly asks women to abnegate natural reproduction. But it also anticipates opposition to the argument. Consequently, Firestone entreats women to at least *consider* the technological options. To be sure, technology can be misused by men, and, consequently, women need to be more involved in scientific research. But the point is that 'artificial reproduction is not inherently dehumanising' and 'at the very least, development of an option should make possible an honest re-examination of the ancient value of motherhood' (ibid.: 225). Firestone's plea that feminists at least consider the possibilities received a mainly hostile reaction in the 1970s and 1980s (see, for example, Arditti *et al.* 1984). She did not continue this particular debate. After suffering a nervous breakdown, she published her account of the journey of mental patients through the US health system in the evocatively titled *Airless Spaces* (Firestone 1998).

While few have fully embraced Firestone's argument, it was to have greater appeal decades on as feminists began to draw attention to the potential of biotechnologies to disrupt conventional notions of parent-hood, identity and the naturalness of 'ordinary' sexual reproduction in ways that could benefit women (e.g. Farquhar 1996; Shildrick 1997). Moreover, her suggestion that reproductive technology can – to use her own term – 'evaporate' the false dichotomy that biology has created between men and women echoes in Donna Haraway's argument that cybertechnology not only opens up the possibility for women to define themselves outside conventional binary categories but sounds the death knell for biological authority itself (1997) (discussed further in Chapter 7). But, in the early 1970s such debates were some time in the future. At that juncture, the gut reaction was to assert that to take woman's natural power to give life away 'is to take away her trump card and to leave her with an empty hand, entirely vulnerable to men's power' (Tong 1998: 71–2).

Like Firestone, Mary O'Brien (1981) conceived of reproduction as the essential material base of human history. She also wished to show, contra Marxism, that male dominance is much more than economic in form. For O'Brien, reproduction is *the* central concern of feminist theory and practice and the subject and object of an integrative philosophy. She urged feminists not to eschew their natural reproductive function but to make it 'the central concern of feminist theory and practice' (ibid.: 92). Responding directly to Firestone and drawing upon her own experience as a midwife, she asserted that childbirth is not inherently barbaric; it is a social and cultural affair – a cultural and social affair that, untrammelled by the distortions of patriarchy, which make hospital birth an occasion presided over by obstet-rical entrepreneurs, is a 'quintessentially social celebration of the strength of being female' (ibid.: 10). O'Brien maintained that birth is much more than the material or biological base of the social relations of production; it is a dialectical process that changes historically. Reproductive conscious-ness was fundamentally altered, for example, when men became aware of physiological paternity and when, with the advent of birth control, women became (at least in theory) able to choose parenthood. In common with many others, she argued that women of the 1970s and early 1980s had become alienated from their bodies, as birth was abstracted from its social context by male-dominated reproductive medicine as it fractured the experi-ence of pregnancy and childbirth into a series of artificially separate moments: the moment of ovulation; the moment of copulation; the moment of conception; the moment of gestation; the moment of labour; the moment of birth, and so on. This fragmentation was seen as intrinsic to the male appropriation of birth by turning it into an abstract medicalised process.

Disputes over 'who controls birth' have been querulous to say the least. Indeed, as the early Firestone–O'Brien debate attests, arguments between feminists have sometimes been as (if not more) heated as those against medicine. Much pivots on the vexed issue of essentialism. In its stronger form, represented by the arguments of Daly, O'Brien and others, women's bodies have been stripped of their biological potential by patriarchy. But there is no pure physical category prior to meaning waiting to be reclaimed, even for these writers. As O'Brien put it, reproductive experience is 'rooted in the dialectical structure of the primordial biological experience of our *lived bodies*' and therefore transformed by history (1981: 44, my emphasis). *Either* we can distort the raw material or potentiality of the female biological body by patriarchal ideologies that construe it as precarious and inefficient, with extremely damaging consequences for women's health, *or* we can cultivate the health-enhancing qualities of women's capacity to reproduce and to give birth without undue or 'unnatural' intervention. The latter, of course, is entrusted to feminism. The problem, as noted earlier, is that making this feminist case always risks essentialism since it evokes difference at every turn. This is most evident in the contrasts that are drawn between 'natural-women controlled' and 'unnatural-male controlled' birth. The principal organising contrast is the male takeover of a female domain, at the heart of which lies the boundary line between normal/natural and abnormal/unnatural birth. It is therefore useful to take a very brief look at the history of 'who controls childbirth', before turning to recent thinking.

Two models of childbirth

Feminists, and others sympathetic to midwifery and natural birth, highlight the authoritative place of midwifery before the male-medical takeover, which began in seventeenth-century Europe (Beckett 2005; Michie and Cahn 1996). The question posed is: if both numerically and in terms of skill, female midwives were far superior to the emerging male-midwife of the 1600s, then how were men able to usurp their domain? The answer lies in the rise of modern 'scientific' medicine and the opportunities that it provided for specialisation. As Roy Porter put it, 'the division of labour was one of the nineteenth-century's big ideas, and it affected medicine no less than other spheres of life' (1997: 381). Before this time there had been little to commend midwifery to men, since it was not 'proper' medicine. The association of childbirth with pollution alone was enough to deter them. Birth was far better left to female midwives who, by dint of their sex, were suited to be the cleaners-up in domestic life (Oakley 1976). By the 1700s, the new respectability of anatomy meant that doctors who specialised in obstetrics could study the structure of the gravid uterus. The discovery of auscultation meant they could listen to the pregnant abdomen. The use of ergotamine to stem post-partum haemorrhage – a major cause of death – and the use of anaesthesia to manage pain provided the possibility of real intervention. The making available of the previously jealously guarded medical forceps in the early eighteenth century was particularly important in promoting the medical management of birth. A major catalyst for change, and a blow to female midwifery in England, came in the 1830s when obstetrics was incorporated into the medical curriculum.

It is possible within this general narrative to construe the development of obstetrics simply as part of the increasing acceptance of doctors in all aspects of health care. But it was not just a change in the management of birth that was at issue but the fact that the new practitioners were men. The man-midwife or accoucher – the forerunner of the modern obstetrician – initially troubled expectations about what was appropriate for men and women. The unacceptability of mixing the sexes, who ought to be distinct, was highlighted, for example, in the bisected figures of mid- to late-nineteenth-century prints (Jordanova 1999). Although the man-midwife on the frontispiece to John Blunt's *Man-Midwife Dissected* (1793) has an aristocratic bearing, the written legend describes him as a monster in his propensity to crudity and indecency. This is represented in the drawing by his dubious use of savage potions and instruments, such as the forceps (a particular worry of Blunt's). The body in the drawing is bisected by a hard vertical line, with the man-midwife on one side and the traditional female-midwife on the other. Although by countering the new developments Blunt seems to be protecting women from the attentions of male medicine, he is actually more concerned with protecting what is natural to women. He made clear that midwifery is really only the superintending of nature and therefore natural women's work. Thus he remarked that the notion of a '*man*-mid*wife* is as absurd as that of *woman*-coach*man*' (ibid.: 61, emphasis in original). Moreover, his text was directed not to pregnant women, but to their husbands in order that they might learn how to counteract, as he put it, this 'national evil'. Blunt's worry, then, was more with the unnaturalness of men's movement into this sphere, which was female by right (or nature), than with the usurpation of a female domain.

But most believed that although birth may have been 'natural to women', it by no means followed that they were equipped to deal with it. As Marjorie Tew explains, obstetrics triumphed through 'captivating bluff and dishonest disparagement' of rival midwives and enticing clients to transfer their custom (1990: 291; see also Donnison 1977). Defamation of their character and denigration of their empirical skill was intrinsic to the de-skilling of midwives, which allowed obstetricians to police the boundaries of practice by claiming the 'abnormal' as their own and confining midwives to the 'normal' (itself constructed as a voluble state). In England, the Midwives Act of 1902 eventually left midwives as independent practitioners in charge of natural births, but with an obligation to call on a medical practitioner if abnormalities arose. The catch, of course, was that definitions of what counts as normal would be in the hands of obstetricians, not midwives.

Obstetrical control over birth was consolidated in the 1920s and 1930s as appeals to safety and women's desire for pain relief provided the opportunity to transfer birth from the home to the hospital. Even though hospitals were not necessarily more safe, they were part of 'the bright new sanitised world of medical science', which made them attractive to women (Symonds and Hunt 1996: 92). In this context, pain seemed a throwback to the 'dark ages'. In England, for example, 70 per cent of births took place in hospital by 1965. By the early 1970s, Dublin obstetrician Kieran O'Driscoll was asserting that 'the permissive attitude to labour is now an anachronism' and assuring every woman that her first baby would be born within twelve hours of labour (O'Driscoll *et al*. 1972: 136). Rigid protocols were applied, such as mandatory intervention by artificial rupture of the membranes and oxytocin infusion if cervical dilation did not exceed one centimetre each hour. In the United States, the so-called Freidman curve – after obstetrician Emanuel Freidman – mapped the ideal evolution of cervical dilation and foetal descent in labour, setting the second stage at 76 minutes for women having their first, and 32 minutes for women having subsequent babies (Freidman 1978). O'Driscoll and colleagues extolled this as turning birth into 'an intensive care situation' (O'Driscoll *et al*. 1972: 135).

By 1970, 100 per cent hospital birth was being recommended in England based on the reported finding that, as the proportion of hospital births increased, the incidence of maternal and infant mortality decreased. But as Tew (1990) explains, this confuses covariance with cause and effect. In the course of teaching her students how much they could learn about various diseases from official statistics, Tew discovered to her 'complete surprise' that routine statistics did not support the widely accepted hypothesis that hospitalisation had *caused* the decline in maternal and infant mortality. On the contrary, her analysis revealed that 'obstetrical intervention rarely improves the natural process' and birth is safer the less the process is interfered with (ibid.: vii). She argued that downward trends are explainable by the gradual spread of prosperity, which means that far fewer women are malnourished and 'reproductively inefficient'.

As Kathryn Beckett remarks, past and present, the idioms of 'the natural' and 'the normal' are best understood as 'part of an effort to contest medical control of birth' (2005: 254). Bolstered by the wider authority of medicine, obstetrics had been able to convince us that the female body was unreliable. The feminist response turned on a distinction between women's understanding of reproduction and that of the (overwhelmingly) male medical profession. Women patients and their (mostly) male doctors were positioned as two different groups with two contrasting perspectives that flow from women's capacity to reproduce and men's desire to control it.

In a landmark paper published in the early 1980s, Hilary Graham and Ann Oakley argued that differences between pregnant women and their doctors go way beyond differences of opinion about approaches and procedures, such as 'whether a pregnancy is normal or pathological or whether or not labour should be routinely induced' to 'a qualitatively different way of looking at the nature, context and management of reproduction' (1981: 51). They argued that women and their doctors differ fundamentally on the nature of childbearing and the context in which it is seen: is pregnancy a natural process integral to women's life experience, or a medical process 'abstracted from the woman's life-experiences and treated as an isolated medical event'? (ibid.: 52). Following on from this, women and doctors differ on their criteria of success. For obstetricians it is limited to the immediate outcome of a physically healthy baby while the woman is in their care, while for women it is so much more and concerns the integration of motherhood into the rest of their life. The final difference concerns how the quality of reproduction is assured, that is, who controls childbearing. How far are women subject to the 'expert' knowledge of obstetricians gained from formal scientific training and how far are they able to employ their own 'individualised and to some extent intuitive knowledge built up from bodily experience?' (ibid.: 55). Graham and Oakley maintained that these differences are revealed in conflicts over the status of reproduction as health or as an illness, over expertise in judging symptoms and their meaning, over who makes decisions about aspects of care, and over the nature of communication between the woman and her doctor. The political agenda is clear: any change *within* the current system of maternity care (such as educating doctors to be less dogmatic about their patients 'needs') will always be limited. Consequently, more radical change may be called for, such as a return to home delivery and a transfer of responsibility from doctors to midwives (ibid.: 54–5).

The distinction between normal, natural, woman-controlled birth on the one hand, and abnormal, technological, male/medical controlled birth on the other was the flashpoint for feminist sociological research on health and remains influential to the present day. Be it the cooler tone of the social scientific monograph or the more heated language of the popular book or activist tract, a common conclusion emerged early on; as the Brighton Women and Science Group put it: 'it is time that we reclaimed our bodies, our childbirth. We must insist on giving birth the way *we* want' (1980: 180, emphasis in the original).

Sociological research quickly began to reflect this position. Diana Scully's influential research had the dual aims of contributing to sociological knowledge on how residents (doctors in training) in obstetrics and gynaecology acquire skill and of empowering women to make changes by demystifying medical knowledge (Scully 1977, 1980, 2003). Finding themselves hungry for surgical experience, residents in Scully's study viewed their patients as a resource through which to learn skills rather than in terms of their personal health needs. She likens the residents' modus operandi to that of a salesman: 'the greater the number of contacts' they had with women, 'the greater the probability of making a sale'. She found that they would 'judge within minutes whether a woman was going to buy a hysterectomy', justifying their aggressive practices on the grounds that female reproductive organs are expendable equipment (Scully 1980: 224). Scully makes recommendations for women, in this instance on how to reduce unnecessary surgery. She advises a move away from professional self-regulation toward consumer involvement and the greater utilisation of non-physician women health workers such as nurse-midwives. Echoing this sentiment, Gena Corea remarks upon the life-changing consequences of her investigations into medical violations against women's civil rights in 1971. She related that at the start 'I was not a feminist. By the time I had finished, the evidence I had gathered forced me to become one.' It is not, she asserts, simply a matter of recognising that women are compelled to receive treatment from 'members of the more powerful sexual caste', but of taking responsibility for their own health – rather than passively handing it over to men – and changing things (Corea 1985: 78, originally published in 1977). The essential ingredients for change were summed up by Ann Oakley as follows: 'an end to unnecessary medical intervention in childbirth; the re-domestication of birth; a return to female-controlled childbirth; and the provision of therapeutic support for women after childbirth' (1980: 295–6). The midwife has been the lynchpin of these developments.

Feminism and midwifery

Social scientists, sociologists included, have found midwifery's feminist credentials in the historical struggle for control over birth briefly described above and in present-day practice, where a natural affinity between women and midwives is often taken to mean that, untrammelled by male obstetrics and oppressive institutional controls, they will work together to achieve a positive birth experience. Thus as Lara Foley and Christopher Faircloth discuss, 'social scientific literature on midwifery has placed a midwife, or a holistic, model of childbirth in polar opposition to a technocratic or medical model' (2003: 165). Sociologist Barbara Katz Rothman dedicated her highly influential book *In Labour. Women and Power in the Birthplace* 'to the midwives, daughters of time'. For Rothman, real life experience – in this instance, of giving birth herself – was the wellspring of sociological insight. She writes, 'in my personal research I had begun to uncover a fascinating lode of data. As a social scientist I was eager to go back and mine it' (Rothman 1982: 23). She paints a stark contrast between what she calls 'medical' and 'midwifery models' of birth: on the one hand, a pellucid 'man's-eye view of women's bodies' reflecting the technological orientation of the late-twentieth century; on the other, an initially more cloudy vision eventually pieced together as the 'midwifery model', which focused and centred on women and saw reproduction in a 'holistic, naturalistic way' (ibid.: 24). The heart of the difference, for Rothman, lies in how the foetus–mother relationship is viewed. Within the patriarchal 'medical model', the foetus is the child of the man in the woman. Since the medical management of pregnancy is understood in terms of the separation of the foetus and the mother, their needs are at odds with each other. The obstetrician must intervene, for example, by using his surgical

scissors to stop the baby from ripping the mother apart, and using forceps
to prevent the mother's body from crushing the baby. By contrast, in the
'midwifery model', mother and foetus are described as 'an organic whole';
meeting the needs of one meets the needs of the other (ibid.: 276). During
labour, the mother works to deliver her baby with the midwife's assistance.
Rothman explains that in her pipe dream she would simply do away with
obstetrics. Should the need for intervention arise, such as the transfer to
a surgeon for a Caesarean section, this would be on the mandate of the
midwife and the woman.

Of course, it is important not to lump all midwives together – they are
a diverse group whose jurisdiction to practise varies considerably from
country to country (and within some countries, such as the US and Canada,
from state to state and province to province). As Tara Kaufmann puts it,
'feminism is not a precondition of midwifery and midwifery is far from
being a feminist profession' (2004: 8). Research by sociologists Deborah
Sullivan and Rose Weitz on lay midwifery in the US back in the early 1980s
makes this clear: only six of their fifty respondents became midwives as a
'consciously feminist response to male-dominated obstetrics' (1988: 79).
And, as Jane Sandall argues, there is no evidence for the assumption that,
because midwifery is a female-dominated occupation it will guard women's
interests and 'give a more holistic, empathetic and egalitarian style of care,
which will ensure choice and control for women' (1999: 358). Along with
others, Sandall points out that policies that stress 'midwifery values' such
as 'continuity of care' can help to carve out discrete spheres of knowledge
and expertise and professional power over other practitioners that are
themselves legitimated by the primacy of the midwife–woman relationship.

But within professional elites in particular, many midwives do self-define
as feminist. The underlying assumption that feminism is pro-midwifery
and midwifery practice is – or certainly should be – feminist informed is
seen, for example, in contractions such as 'midwifery feminism' (Stephens
2004) or 'feminist midwifery' (Campbell and Porter 1997), used by midwives
and by social scientists alike. Nicky Leap explains that feminism and
midwifery have been entwined in her life since she came to midwifery via
the women's liberation movement as a student in the 1970s. She remarks
that in those days 'feminism was easily identified as integral to midwifery
practice' (Leap 2004: 198). Writing in the late 1980s, nurse-midwives
William and Sandi McCool (1989) endorse this point and lament that not
all midwives recognise or wish to embrace feminism. Many midwife-
academics share these concerns, believing that since the hegemonic power
of the medical model of birth actively obscures the natural affinity between
midwifery and feminism, there is a need actively to convince colleagues of
what feminism has to offer. Mavis Kirkham, for example, explains that
'the word "midwife" seems to me to mean in concrete terms exactly what
"feminist" means ideologically: with woman' (1986: 35; see also Trego
2005). Equally, in a foreword to a collection on feminist perspectives on

pregnancy, birth and maternity care for midwives, Sheila Hunt remarks that 'in due course no-one will attempt to define midwifery without acknowledging the feminist "way of seeing". Only then we will move confidently to woman-centred care and really mean it' (2004: ix-x).

A critical reflection

(Female) midwifery's struggle with (male) obstetrics and its consequences for women's health have become central tropes in a much wider political project founded on a binary distinction between the male and female body and male and female ways of being in the world (Annandale and Clark 1996, 1997). The (biological) sex/(social) gender distinction has been employed to argue that, since social oppression occurs through the denigration and patriarchal control of women's bodies, the route to better health and health care lies in a re-valuing of women's bodies and promoting women-controlled or woman-centred alternatives. This has underwritten a series of quite obdurate matched oppositions: on the one hand, birth that is natural, midwife-led and woman-centred; on the other, birth that is technological, male-controlled and obstetric-led.

This is not to say that midwife researchers and sociologists are doggedly unreflexive in their use of the contrast; indeed, it is noticeable that they have begun to problematise it in recent years (see, for example, Kent 2000; Walsh 2004). It is also apparent that the rather stark polarisations of the 1970s and early 1980s generally have given way to more subtle contrasts. Commentators are far less likely, for example, to appeal to a past 'golden age' of childbirth to support present claims that birth is inherently fulfilling and largely trouble-free when released from the grip of male obstetrics. There is far more recognition that, in common with other aspects of health and health care, birth is socially and politically laden and that it cannot exist in any essential way outside this. It is increasingly appreciated, as Barbara Katz Rothman (1981) put it some time ago now, that the notion of natural birth is a slippery concept. At least in theory it is possible to make a distinction, as Rothman does, between 'natural' and 'prepared' childbirth, the latter referring to the instinctual and untamed and the former to the use of techniques to 'cope with', 'get through' or to achieve the 'right' birth experience. But, as noted earlier, it is questionable whether the former can ever be a reality. As Becky Mansfield (2008) discusses, it is social practices that allow childbirth to be natural. Thus practices that might be construed as 'natural' can also be interpreted as 'interventions' – if by interventions we mean not letting nature take its course unfettered (whatever that might be) – such as adopting one birth position rather than another that might be 'naturally' preferred, moving around when one might 'naturally' prefer to be still, or inducing birth by a combination of castor oil, enema and a warm bath to 'speed' labour in order to achieve a desired birth experience. In some instances women and midwives engage in these practices in order to meet the expectations of powerful outsiders. For example, attempts might be made to speed up a labour deemed to be too lengthy and thereby 'dangerous' by male partners, family members or obstetricians. But equally these practices might be consciously engaged in to create what has been socially defined as a 'natural birth' (Annandale 1988; Mansfield 2008).

Even so, circumspection still tends to be a precursor to spelling out, rather than to relinquishing, the contrast. It is still fairly unusual for feminist and feminist-informed commentators not to begin by alluding, critically or otherwise, to 'two models' or 'competing perspectives' on birth. Contrasts therefore linger in the feminist and other imaginaries and inform discussion, albeit in more astute and nuanced ways. So even where oppositional language is questioned, distinctions tend to run through the ensuing discussion. For example, Ann Oakley regrets that we have become trapped within a misleading language of opposition between, on the one hand, 'midwives, women, health, normality and so forth' and, on the other, 'obstetricians, disease, abnormality, science' (1989: 215). She challenges this by arguing, in the manner discussed earlier, that it was set up in the first place by male 'science' to denigrate midwives as unreliable and even downright devious individuals. She then turns male 'science' back on itself by showing that it is hardly scientific. With its frequent and routine use of potentially harmful practices, such as electronic foetal heart rate monitoring, high rates of the induction of labour and Caesarean sections, she remarks that obstetrics is neither 'effective nor safe' (ibid.: 217). Appropriating the quintessentially scientific method – the controlled trial – Oakley draws on the existing evidence (which she recognises is limited) to argue that midwives' caring and social support – in short, love – is far more safe and effective. Ultimately, both Oakley's critique and her concluding position rest far more on engaging the language of opposition than in dismantling it.

Social anthropologist and birth activist Sheila Kitzinger is convinced that women 'all over the world share the intense experience of birth in similar ways, and that we have the innate and expert skills to give birth perfectly' (2004: 16). This premise from the re-edition (with a new introductory essay) of her book *The Experience of Childbirth* (2004, originally published in 1962), rests on a juxtaposition of natural birth and birth as a medical event. Despite an appeal to women's own 'innate' and 'expert skills', there is an abiding sense that birth is something that needs to be consciously worked for. As Becky Mansfield shows in her (2008) analysis of representations of natural birth in books written for a popular readership, this is far from unique. Kitzinger's book is a fund of information on the techniques that women can learn for birth. Thus there are complex and detailed exercises on how to relax to help a woman 'relate herself better to her body' (Kitzinger 2004: 97), including twelve ways of 'exploring release over different parts of the body' and instructions on how to breathe in labour (ibid.: 115). On the latter, Kitzinger remarks:

it might be thought that we could safely leave breathing to chance, and that most women in labour breathe all right anyway. But women in labour frequently flush out too much carbon dioxide from their bloodstream with a resulting reduction in the flow of blood to the baby.

(ibid.: 115)

She explains that women need to harmonise the way they breathe with the rhythm of labour. Consequently, four exercises are provided to help them learn: 'deep thoracic breathing', 'upper thoracic breathing', 'mouth-centred breathing' and 'diaphragmatic breathing'. By stressing the need for these techniques, Kitzinger challenges the foundations of her own argument, for how can women be natural experts in their own bodies and also need such detailed technical instruction?

This suggests that it may be as difficult to work with the binary contrasts that flow from the sex/gender distinction as it is to question them. The reason for this is that concepts such as 'natural birth' and 'woman-controlled birth' are referential. When the sex (biology)/gender (social) distinction is employed, natural birth and related concepts tend to take on essential meanings that cannot actually be sustained. Just as the notion of 'working class' makes little sense except in relation to 'middle class' (and vice versa), natural and non-natural/technological birth acquire their meaning only through ongoing dialogue with each other. Each concept is controvertible, meaningful only in terms of a shifting relationship with its imputed opposites. From this vantage point it is not surprising that the enjoining of midwifery with feminism can be marshalled to quite different ends. According to the *Concise Oxford English Dictionary*, the term midwife comes from the middle English 'mid' (with) and 'wife' (in the archaic sense, woman). Rich with meaning, the notion of being 'with woman' is apt to be drawn into the service of legitimating quite different versions of midwifery practice. Take, for example, Meg Taylor's (2000) appeal to a set of difficult to articulate but intuitive core 'midwifery values'. She makes clear that not all who practise under the name are 'true' midwives and that 'true' midwifery skills are lost when midwives practise unthinkingly within the system as nurse-midwives or obstetric nurses. Only if they practise midwifery rather than obstetric nursing are midwives practising feminism. Carrie Klima (2001: 93) makes much the same claim, writing as a certified nurse-midwife, that is, from 'within the system' in Taylor's terms.

It is therefore difficult to work with any ease within the binaries of the 'two models' or 'competing perspectives' because they are themselves chronically unstable rather than essential givens. As Paula Treichler explains, we cannot look for what childbirth really *is* in the discourse of its various protagonists. A counter discourse 'does not arise as a pure autonomous radical language embodying the purity of a new politics' (Treichler 1990: 132). It is not a pre-determined starting point for struggle, but an outcome of struggle, 'an unstable, negotiated, and often quite temporary cultural prescription' (ibid.: 133). This is not to suggest that contrasts should not be strategically drawn upon; indeed, there may be compelling political reasons to do so. However unstable definitions may be, when embodied in policies and everyday practices they have real material powers, and counterpoints are important (Beckett 2005). But we still need to be aware that 'essence *as* irreducible has been *constructed* to be irreducible' (Fuss 1989: 4, emphasis in the original). Failure to appreciate this risks locking women into 'natural' reproductive roles on the basis of their difference from men. Ironically, feminists can then find it as difficult to think beyond the female reproductive body as (male) biomedicine. And, moreover, they risk 'a series of deeply problematic ties between women and nature' that evoke 'natural femininity' (Michie and Cahn 1996). There is a marked tendency, for example, to see all women as potential mothers. Thus as Julie Kent points out, despite recognising that motherhood has been romanticised and idealised, Sheila Kitzinger still seems to essentialise women. Kent aptly remarks that in Kitzinger's perspective, the 'universality of motherhood seems to return to a biological or maternal instinct just at the point when "culture" takes effect' (2000: 111). Thus it might be argued that the passage of time has actually meant relatively little in terms of developing an effective challenge to the assumptions of normative maternity that early sociological research on reproduction sought to contest (referred to earlier in the chapter). Moreover, as Lynda Layne discusses, portraying birth as 'a natural womanly talent' obscures from view all those 'women for whom pregnancy and birth do not come easy, if at all' (2003: 1888–9; see also Michie and Cahn 1996).

Conclusions

The purpose of this and the preceding chapter has been to chart the two research directions – one broadly associated with 'equality feminism', the other with 'difference feminism' – that grew out of feminists' engagement with the sex (biology)/gender (social) distinction. Each generated an inspirational, agenda-setting body of research that has travelled in time and remains influential today. However, each brought problems in its wake. With its overwhelming emphasis on the *social* nature of women's oppression, equality feminism has sought to explain women's health status largely without reference to the biological body and in relation to women's social roles and statuses, largely outside the wider social relations of gender. In contrast, 'difference feminism' has made the *biological* body not only central to an exploration of women's reproductive well-being but also vital to the analysis of their wider oppression. So broadly speaking, research on health status has floundered because of its tendency to collapse the biological into the social and research on reproductive health has floundered because of the opposite tendency of collapsing the social into the biological. This is not to propose that the latter has been crudely essentialist. In most research it is the body's raw material or biological potential that matters: depending on social context this potential can either be allowed to flourish, thus contributing to women's well-being, or it can be undermined, to the detriment of their health. However, this body of research always risks essentialism in its tendency to evoke difference at every turn. This is most evident in the obdurate contrasts between 'natural–women controlled' and 'unnatural–male controlled' birth.

By the late 1980s, feminists were drawing ever more attention to the problems that flow from the privileging of difference – be it biological or social – in the sex/gender distinction. The next chapter reflects critically on the limitations of the sex/gender distinction as a basis for a feminist understanding of women's health through a critical engagement with recent feminist theory.

5 Thinking again about sex, gender and health

Introduction

In Chapter 2, I argued that research on women's health has been shaped by the constellation of factors that orbit the powerful sex (biology)/gender (social) distinction. At this point it may be useful to sum up the main arguments that have been made in this respect so far. We have seen that in contexts where women's biological bodies have been negatively defined – which marks out most of history – the equation of men and the social, women and the biological has been a fundamental tool for the oppression of women. The sex/gender distinction was a powerful counter-framework and a veritable treasure trove for research on women's health. But it harboured considerable problems that came to light as research progressed. One of these was a bifurcated agenda, with a tendency to focus on either the social or the biological. Another related problem, touched upon in the preceding chapters but taken up further here, is the focus on male/female difference. As discussed in Chapter 2, when sociological research on health was developing during the 1960s and 1970s, differences between male and female experience, or the bi-polar social script, were a palpable feature of society. It is not surprising that this prompted a search for the factors that differentiate male/female health status and their experience of health and health care. The current chapter focuses on the problems that this poses for the analysis of health.

Differentiation

Since ultimately their 'biological sex' is the only characteristic that all women can share – even though they do not necessarily do so – it has become an obdurate marker of distinction. In theory, 'social gender' is more open than biological sex – sex, it has been argued, is the constant, gender the variable – but in practice, feminists have tended to divide and distinguish men and women on social (gender) grounds as much as they have along (sex) biological lines. As we saw in Chapter 3, this has been apparent in research on the social determinants of health status. At the same time as it is taken as read that men and women are not intrinsically different – since gender, so it goes, is not tied to sex – assumptions typically have been made about *which* social factors are relevant for male experience and *which* for female experience, in advance of research. Research gets trapped in the ideological context of what it is trying to analyse (Carrigan *et al.* 1987) as difference is sought from the outset. As Christine Di Stefano explains outside the context of health, feminist analysis appears to have 'undone one version of a presumably basic difference, thought to be rooted in nature, and come up with another, albeit more debatably basic than the previous one' (1990: 64). Even when the same overall questions are posed about men's and women's health (and until quite recently conjoint research has been rare), results are often read through the lens of differences rather than similarities (Annandale 1998a, 1998b). Indeed, as also noted in Chapter 3, difference has been so deep-seated that sometimes similarities do not get reported at all (Kandrack *et al.* 1991; Macintyre *et al.* 1996). Although she is not referring to health, Linda Nicholson argues that the physiological self is still viewed as 'the "given" on which characteristics are "superimposed"; it provides the location for establishing where specific social influences are to go' (1999: 55). She dubs this the 'coat rack' view of self-identity: the biological body is viewed as a type of rack upon which different cultural artefacts, especially those of personality and behaviour, are placed. While this is not necessarily determinist, it does imply a biological foundationalism (Nicholson 1994).

Protectionist policies

The focus on difference is an understandable reaction to medical and social research, which has a long and ingrained history of making women invisible by privileging men (Rapp 2001). Women's exclusion was justified historically on the grounds of protection. A raft of protectionist policies followed the Nuremberg Code of 1949, which outlined the basic moral, ethical and legal requirements of research with human subjects. A series of tragic incidents such as thalidomide and diethylstilbestrol (DES), alongside the exposure of unethical research practice such as the Tuskegee syphilis and Holmesburg prison experiments (Hornblum 1998; Jones 1981), spurred stringent regulations in the US Department of Health and Human Services (Wizemann and Pardue 2001). Although policy guidelines did not exclude specific populations, they did state that vulnerable subjects must not be exploited. Consequently, researchers became averse to including women in their studies given the risks to those who became pregnant and potentially vulnerable during drug-related research. Protectionist policy pertained until 1990, when a landmark Government Accounting Office (GAO) report to Congress documented the failure of the National Institutes of Health to implement the recommendations of the 1985 US Public Health Task Force on Women's Health Issues, which stated that 'biomedical and behavioural research should be expanded to ensure emphasis on conditions and disease unique to, or more prevalent in, women in all age groups' (GAO, quoted in Eckman 1998: 131). Subsequently the newly created US Office of Research on Women's Health issued statutory guidelines for the inclusion of women in research. Of course, this is not bound to ensure that they are given equal attention (Plechner 2000). Social epidemiological research, for example, has a marked tendency to obscure women's (and also men's) presence either by aggregating data or routinely adjusting for sex (Doyal 2003; Inhorn and Whittle 2001; Kaufert 1999; Wizemann and Pardue 2001).

Clinical and social epidemiological researchers alike typically have taken the male body and male experience as the 'gold standard' for the population as a whole, assuming – if it is thought about at all – that this is generalisable to women. This continues to this day, but it was during the 1970s that female researchers first began to open up what has been dubbed the 'black box' of medical science, to 'poke around in its interior, look for women, and ask "who hid them, how and why?"' (Kaufert 1999: 120). The negative consequences of taking men as the norm are not difficult to discern. In studies of population health, it leads to a neglect of how determinants of health may be different for women and men, and in the delivery of health care, it runs the risk of making assumptions that certain diseases 'belong' to men and, consequently, of misdiagnosing signs and symptoms in women. For example, CHD, the single largest cause of death for women in most western countries, was severely under-researched until very recently because it has been defined as a male disease (Bird and Rieker 2008; Emslie 2005; Emslie *et al.* 2001). Clinical and lay perceptions of the disease continue to be heavily clouded by the later onset in women (typically by seven to ten years and associated with the protective advantage of oestrogen before menopause) and by lingering and inaccurate stereotypes of the 'coronary candidate' among the general population that heart disease results from the stresses that middle-class men experience in the workplace (Riska and Heikell 2007). There is now accumulated evidence that physicians are less likely to recognise the clinical signs of CHD in women and less likely to refer them for diagnostic tests, such as angiography and procedures such as arteriography and bypass surgery (see, for example, Arber *et al.* 2006; Shaw *et al.* 2004). The male image of CHD clearly reflects the 'coat rack' model of the body and identity (Nicholson 1999: 55) referred to earlier: certain traits – such as the drive, impatience and competitiveness of the so-called 'type A' personality – are characterised as male and, consequently, it is male bodies that are identified as 'at risk'. As Elianne Riska discusses, this image is not only 'gendered' but also class and time bound, reflecting many of the 'values and behaviours that were crucial parts of white middle-class masculinity in the 1950s and 1960s' (2004: 18).

The response of feminism to the exclusion or invisible presence of women in clinical and epidemiological research has been to invert the focus on men in favour of a focus on women and, in so doing, to highlight difference. This has involved bringing female-specific health issues such as pregnancy and childbirth to the fore and highlighting the specificity of women's experience of 'shared' health problems such as heart disease, that is, making clear that women's health is about more than their reproductive organs. While this has the considerable merit of unmasking the suppositions of male-dominated medical research and practice discussed above, it also has downsides. Not the least of these is foreclosing criticism of developments such as gender-specific medicine.

Gender-specific medicine

Gender-specific medicine is rapidly growing in influence as observed in publications, international conferences and meetings, research and health care centres. Three of the most well-known centres are the Partnership for Gender-specific Medicine at Columbia University in the US, the Centre for Gender Medicine at the Karolinska Institute in Stockholm, Sweden, and the Centre for Gender in Medicine at Charité Universitätsmedzin in Berlin, Germany. On the face of it, the use of the term gender in 'gender-specific' medicine is simply a misnomer, since it would appear that what is really meant is 'biological sex'. Yet advocates of gender-specific medicine make claims to be continuing the agenda of the women's health movement and evoke the sex (biology)/gender (social) distinction. For example, leading proponent Marianne Legato MD remarks:

> before any discussion about the differences between men and women, one must make a distinction between what is the consequence of biologic sex, and what is the result of the larger phenomenon of the impact of a culture or society on the biologic male or female.
>
> (2003b: 923)

Legato's vision is for a future where 'all doctors will be gender-specific doctors, who treat men and women more accurately and more effectively, and who above all are more cognizant of the complexity of what it means to be a male or a female' (Legato 2003a: 241). Yet the new discipline of gender-specific medicine is defined in a very limited way as 'the science of the differences in the normal physiology of men and women and of the way they experience disease' (Legato 2003b: 917). And this is what makes its growth particularly concerning: it provides a 'strong mandate and agenda for research on sex differences understood strictly in biological terms to proliferate' (Grace 2007: 4).

So it is not simply that sex is a synonym for gender, but that gender, or the socio-cultural, ceases to matter. This is highlighted by Antje Kampf (2006) who reports that most papers presented at the first worldwide symposium on gender-specific medicine, in Berlin 2006 (the Berlin Symposium), were predicated on the notion that biological influences precede cultural and social influences. Similarly, although the spearhead publication from the US Institute of Medicine, *Exploring the Biological Contributions to Human Health. Does Sex Matter?* (Wizemann and Pardue 2001), 'focuses on the effects of biological sex differences on health and the need to evaluate these biological differences in every study, it does not fully examine how these biological factors interact with social and cultural factors' (Bird and Rieker 2008: 227). In the gender-specific paradigm more generally, where 'social' or 'cultural' factors are referred to, they are either so vague as to be virtually meaningless or framed in a highly individualised manner (e.g. personal attitudes or the choices that individuals make about their health). The social therefore becomes a residual category that is devoid of meaning and unrelated to the wider social structural factors that impinge on health.

Moreover, it is not only that, more often than not, discussion proceeds by reference to biology but that it proceeds by reference to biological *difference* (Grace 2007; Kampf 2006). Thus, as Victoria Grace writes, 'the pendulum is swinging away from an era of erasure of difference within medicine and its emphasis on sameness (with the problems of male-as-norm), towards an era of valorising the significance of sex difference' (2007: 5). Why is this happening? To answer this question we first of all need to take note of the heavy emphasis on specific diseases or health conditions. Diseases of particular parts of the body such as the heart (many of the leading proponents of gender-specific medicine are cardiologists), the bones, the breast, the lungs and the colon are the major focus. As Anne Eckman discusses, the lack of attention to heart attacks in women 'has functioned as a proxy index of medical bias against women' (1998: 138). But more than this, 'the lack of biomedical research about women has also functioned to produce a new narrative about the source of women's inequality – a narrative that foregrounds the need for medicine to embrace a new view of women's bodies' (ibid.: 138). The overriding message of this narrative is that we are missing knowledge about *bits* of their bodies. With this, the 'whole woman' disappears from view along with any interest in the social structural sources of inequality that influence women's health, such as poverty, interpersonal violence and lack of access to resources. Social inequalities are elided through the imagery of women's bodies as 'equal and opposite to a man's' (ibid.: 148).

To complete the answer to the question of why biological difference is valorised, we need to reflect on medicine as a business. Unsurprisingly, given the focus on particular diseases and parts of the body, much of gender-specific medicine is hospital based (including laboratory-based research on the cellular structure of the body) and high-tech in orientation. Corporate partnerships are not uncommon. The Partnership for Gender-specific Medicine at Columbia University in the US, for example, lists current and past supporters such as pharmaceutical companies Procter & Gamble, Wyeth, Bristol-Myers Squibb, Kos Pharmaceuticals, Pfizer, Astra-Zeneca, Johnson and Johnson and CVS/pharmacy (see http://partnership.

hs.columbia.edu/sponsors.html). This continues a history of heavy invest-
ment of the pharmaceutical industry in 'women's health' research, such as
menopausal symptoms (Lagro-Janssen 2007). Even though it is not the
focus of discussion here, it should be noted that gender-specific medicine
concerns men as much as it does women. For example, the *Journal of
Men's Health and Gender,* which endorses gender-specific medicine, contains
a staple diet of articles on the andropause and erectile dysfunction. Sex
differences research therefore has big business potential as discoveries of
'gender-specific' responses to pathogens open up new markets for 'gender-
specific' treatments, such as drug therapies and modes of care. Grace
(2007) provides an illustration of this from a paper presented at the Berlin
Symposium. She recounts the speaker's interest in 'gender pharmacogenomic
clocks', which, it was claimed, would lead to the creation of a biotechnology that provides 'gender time-mapped pharmacogenomic personalised
medicine' (Bendayan quoted in Grace 2007: 8). The promotion of genetic-
and molecular-level research signals the resurgence of biological and genetic
essentialism in the wake of the Human Genome Project (Kampf 2006).
Insufficiently documented or spurious claims of sex-related differences in
genetic associations in diseases are growing (Patsopoulos *et al.* 2007) As
Peter Conrad remarks, the biotechnology industry 'promises a genomic,
pharmaceutical, and technological future that may revolutionalise healthcare'
(2007: 15). Gender-specific medicine looks set to be a major part of this
future.[1]

So far I have argued that although 'social gender' appears, in both conceptual and empirical terms, to be more variable and flexible than 'biological
sex', in actuality it is drawn towards opposition. Recent developments,
such as gender-specific medicine, only serve to reinforce this. This is part
of what Anne Fausto-Sterling calls the 'spreading oil-spill of sex' (2005:
195) and, as noted in Chapter 3, a stark warning sign that biology needs
to be brought back into the feminist fold. The question is, how?

The sex/gender 'looping process'

As we saw in the preceding two chapters, most research has tended either
to positively revalue women's (given) biological difference from men or to
turn biology aside. In both cases, it remains a given. When left as a natural
and fixed dichotomy, sex/biology is highly likely to inform the experience
of social gender; that is, gender is still read through sex (Moi 1999). Raia
Prokhovnik explains that 'as long as gender only trades on a foundational
"natural" sex difference (which undermines an effective difference between
the two terms), then all the elements of the sex/gender distinction are
determined, either biologically or socially or both' (1999: 127). Instead of
liberating women, their oppression can be perpetuated and sometimes even
intensified. Gender built on sex becomes binary difference, too, as 'differences among women are silenced and difference between men and women

privileged; the sameness among women is presumed and the similarity between men and women denied' (Eisenstein 1988: 3).

As discussed in Chapter 1, as fundamental and linked oppositions, sex and gender underwrite further dichotomies such as nature/culture, mind/body and reason/emotion. The clusters that arise are well documented: men are rational, women are irrational; women are associated with nature/body, men with culture/mind, and so on. These oppositions are interdependent since each term derives its meaning from an established contrast, rather than from some intrinsic or pure antithesis. Moreover, as many have pointed out, they are inherently patriarchal given that their 'very structure is privileged by the male/non-male distinction' (Grosz 1990: 101), where the leading term is accorded a primacy that is passed off as 'natural-eternal' (Cixous and Clément 1986: 65) and its opposite is given a subordinate or secondary status. Woman is 'positioned as man's attenuated inversion, as a mere specular reflection through which his identity is grounded' (Kirby 1997: 67). Heterosexist bias is also evident, since everything outside the binary is defined as an anomaly or perversion (de Lauretis 1987; Fuss 1991; Jackson 1999; Mathieu 1996).

Although it is unusual within feminism to apply these general points to health, it is apparent when we do that health and illness are drawn towards opposition, as the biological difference that girds our thinking spills over into the social as a series of new dichotomies are layered one on top of the other. The unfortunate consequence of this binary logic is that positively associated health becomes attached to men, and negatively valued illness to women. It then becomes difficult to see men as ill and women as well. The ironic consequence is that feminism can end up entrenching women's ill health, unintentionally colluding with patriarchy by not letting them be well, that is, pathologising their health. And, of course, as a corollary, construed as well by comparison, it is difficult for men to be ill (Annandale and Clark 1996). In these terms, it is fairly easy to see why men – viewed as strong, resilient, robust and, above all, healthy – are selected into privileged positions and why women are not. Any attempt to undermine patriarchy through social and/or biological difference can be wrong-footed since it gets trapped within the problematic that it is trying to challenge.

This discussion suggests that attempts to challenge patriarchy by distinguishing (biological) sex from (social) gender are problematic. This is because they leave biological sex as difference precisely in order to construe gender as more fluid. Left unchallenged, biological sex remains a binary either/or difference between male and female bodies. Gender ultimately lapses back onto this dichotomy rather than flowing free from it, and hence sex difference continues to be the basis of gendered experience. This means that, although on the surface a lot of feminist research on health has cast biology aside in favour of a focus on social variations between men and women – and, as discussed in Chapter 3, this is a problematic move in itself – it makes a spectral return. An unspoken biological difference is embedded within its framework: social gender is still wedded to biological sex, and both tend to operate in a dichotomous manner.

Since sex has been identified as the culprit in the failure of gender to free women from patriarchal control, it makes sense to challenge the way that it is conceived. It is fairly common now to see the argument that sex is neither natural nor fixed. Erving Goffman (1979) and others made it clear that 'gender attribution' and 'gender display' are ongoing practical accomplishments of everyday life; that is, it has been appreciated for some time that the body is bounded and marked as sexed because we view it through the various social lenses of gender. Christine Delphy puts this well: 'when we connect gender and sex, are we comparing something social with something natural, or are we comparing something social with something which is *also* social (in this case, the way a given society represents "biology" to itself)?' (1993: 5). In these terms, sex is the retrospective projection of gender; gender comes *before* sex, rather than the other way round (Butler 1990, 2004; Elam 1994). This is not to suggest that the material body is a fiction, but rather that sex is the embodiment of gender, although for some feminists, such as Drucilla Cornell (1991), what we perceive as reality (here a sexed body) is quite literally a reality *effect*, produced by the language of gender. Crucially, then, a feedback loop is in operation whereby our ideas about (social) gender are constrained by our limited ability to envisage sex (biology) in anything but dichotomous ways, and the possibility of breaking away from dichotomous perceptions of sex (biology) is restricted by the firm grip that our ideas about social gender as dichotomy have on the biological imagination. This 'looping process' also makes clear that the social need be no more (or less) malleable than the biological.

Feminist biologists and others have pointed out that 'gendered dichotomies are etched deep into the narratives of biology' (Birke 1999: 41; see also Epstein 1990). Perforce nature has been read in highly gendered ways. This is evident in the surge of interest in gender-specific medicine, discussed earlier, which 'endorses the dichotomising and this essentialising of biological sex . . . and disavows attempts to re-theorise biology in non-dualistic terms' (Grace 2007: 7). In gender-specific medicine and more widely, two fixed and dichotomous groups – men and women – are constructed (through the language of sex difference) out of a series of biological and social markers such as hormones and percentage body fat that, in actuality, are best viewed as continua rather than distinctions. As Lynda Birke discusses:

> it does not really matter that scientists themselves would not claim one hormone or other as belonging only to one sex. By *labelling* them as such, a binary narrative is created, which in turn gains currency in the wider culture precisely because it fits so neatly with cultural stereotypes.
>
> (Birke 2000: 592–2; emphasis in original;
> see also Oudshoorn 1994)

Barbara Hanson (2000) likens the tendency to create a dichotomy out of physical characteristics that exist on a continuum to the process of dividing mercury with a ruler. Since the dichotomisation is empirically false – the phenomena reconstitute themselves when the ruler is removed – research findings are distorted. We then take it as read that the constructed male/female difference on the physical attribute in question is important for the aspect of health under consideration, when it may not be. Dichotomous thinking that took hold during the 1800s (Laqueur 1990) therefore has shown an amazing resilience, retaining its grip on biomedical thinking in the face of mounting evidence that the 'defining features' of sex difference, such as the chromosomal 'gold standard', may not be relevant. Hormone levels, for example, can be manipulated with drugs to promote the development of more marked sex attributes and even 'opposite' sex attributes. Yet the will to mark difference persists. Thus the commitment to sexual dimorphism leads to the quite literal carving of difference onto the body in the case of surgical management of intersex (Butler 2004; Kessler 1990, 1998). Functional reproductive capacity is often taken as the divide between men and women. But this in itself is a normative ideal, since at any one point in time, and for the majority of their lives, most females are incapable of reproduction – being, for instance, too old, too young, too malnourished, at the wrong point in their menstrual cycle and so on to 'reproduce' (Cealey Harrison and Hood-Williams 2002).

The fusion of sex and gender therefore is tighter than feminists initially appreciated. The 'looping process' is so entrenched that the grip of patriarchy on women's experience cannot be broken by prising the two apart and stressing the social nature of gender. By implication, then, gender can only fulfil its initial feminist promise and be truly variable – that is, no longer annexed in specific ways with either men or women – when it is no longer tightly bound to sex (biology) as a fixed dichotomy. The logical corollary is a two-headed offence that recasts *both* sex *and* gender as malleable and multiple. This calls for a more porous model of sex/gender, such as that advanced by feminist philosopher Tina Chanter, who is of the opinion that we should be developing a theoretical position whereby 'neither category is evacuated of meaning but both are constituted, in relation to one another, as permeable and instable' (2000: 1240).

This evokes Jacques Derrida's (1982) insistence that dualisms such as male/female and health/illness be re-conceptualised as a cohabitation of terms rather than an oppositional either/or. Here, the object is to resist closure (Linstead 1993) not just by elevating the suppressed term but by subverting or destabilising the hierarchical division itself, so that when thinking of women and men, commonalties become as important as differences and men can no longer be associated with all that is valued and women with all that is devalued (Barrett and Phillips 1992). Arguably it is more difficult to associate men with positive health and women with negative health when sex and gender are *both* conceived as more fluid. This does not mean that difference is of necessity obliterated (in thought or in practice). At the very least, some minimal point of commonality and continuity of debate necessitates the linguistic retention of the familiar terms, 'man' and 'woman' (Fuss 1989: 4). But, more importantly, however much we may fear 'being discovered unwittingly behind enemy lines; caught in the suffocating menace of that carnal envelope' (Kirby 1997: 73), keeping difference in play may have strategic or interventionary value. As we will see in Chapters 6 and 7, it is the artefact against which more fluid and shifting differences of sex/gender are counterposed. In these terms, it is questionable whether it is possible to open up the space for suppressed heterogeneity without evoking the (appearance of) unity (Flax 1990).

From this perspective there is no way of going back to the (mythical) artless biology of patriarchy. It has not simply been uncovered as sexist; it has been undone. The emphasis on fluidity and flow shares the desire of feminist biologists and social science commentators on biology to 'think about the body as process(es) rather than fixed' (Birke 2003: 46). Emphasis is placed on the development of the organism in interaction with the world (rather from some blueprint in the DNA). As Toine Lagro-Janssen puts it, 'a biological organism such as the human body is an open system that is influenced by environmental and evolutionary factors. Genes and sex hormones can never be the only explanations for differences between the sexes' (2007: 12; see also Grosz 1994). Genetic activity is not pre-programmed; it 'guides development by responding to external signals reaching specific cells at specific times' (Fausto-Sterling 2003: 128). Bodies have agency in relation to their environment as they constantly respond to change, both inside and out. Although it is something of a sociological commonplace nowadays to assert that the biological body is socially inscribed, in concrete terms our understanding of this process is very much in its infancy (Birke 1999). Anne Fausto-Sterling marshals her thoughts under the rubric of 'development systems theory' (DST). As she puts it, from the point of view of DST, 'neither naked sex nor naked gender exist. Findings of so-called biological difference do not imply a claim of immutability or inevitability' (Fausto-Sterling 2003: 125). She gives the example of the alleged sex differences in verbal and spatial differences in the part of the brain called the corpus callosum. As she puts it, the assertion of difference is just a starting point; the interesting question is how any differences developed in the first place. Thus, 'what childhood experiences and behaviours contribute to the developing anatomy of the brain? ... How do nerve cells translate externally generated information into specific growth patterns and neural circuits?' (ibid.: 125). In other words, sex and gender are mutually constructed; 'we *acquire* a body rather than a passive unfolding of some preformed blueprint' (ibid.: 131, emphasis in original).

1950s. As activists 'describe every fear, every possible horror suffered at the hands of men, the image they project is one of helplessness and passivity' (ibid.: 44). The message they put across, she claims, is not only one of stifling ever present danger but one of women as fragile and innocent, their bodies chaste objects ever vulnerable to male corruption. Roiphe warns that denial of sexual agency in contemporary feminism backs women into old corners, since it leaves them chasing the very same stereotypes that earlier feminists spent so much time running away from.

It is arguably a short step from questioning feminism's contemporary relevance in this way to the view that feminism itself is guilty not only of holding women back, as Wolf and Roiphe contend, but for all kinds of problems faced by women today. It is also inherently conservative (Archer Mann and Huffman 2005; Heywood and Drake 1997). For Ann Oakley (1998; see also Oakley 2002), these writings are themselves part of the wider backlash against feminism. The backlash that emerged in the 1980s and continues apace today trades on the premise that women may very well be (more) equal, but look where it has got them – they may have greater access to financially and personally rewarding jobs, but is it really worth the mental distress that it causes as they attempt to balance home and working life in an attempt to 'have it all'? (Faludi 1991). Lest it should be concluded that this line of argument is promoted only by younger women, Alison Wolf (2006), a professor at Kings College London, cautions that the emergence of a cadre of 'elite' (well educated, 'high flying') women in professional jobs is extremely damaging for society. Returning us to essentialist notions, she bemoans the decline of what she calls 'female altruism', which has deflected women's attentions from female concerns, such as caring for the family and the sick, which they all once shared.

Disavowing the collective category 'woman', then, might be said to concur with the increasingly popular opinion that gender, and by extension feminism, no longer matters. Many commentators are of the opinion that an emphasis on fluidity and heterogeneity unproblematically endorses individualism at the expense of the shared identity that 'second wave' feminists deem necessary for political action. Thus in Mary Daly's (1993) view, women are living in an age of dismemberment, split from their selves and their connections with others, and feminists are doing precious little to counteract this. As Lynda Birke writes:

> to judge by the titles of many books on the theme, [the body] seems endlessly malleable. It can be 'volatile' or 'flexible', it can be 'leaky', it can be 'slender', it can be 'rejected' or 'deviant'. Upon its surface we can etch the cultural angst of the West.
>
> (Birke 1999: 135)

The body 'is always superficially transformable' (ibid.: 138). Moreover the 'postmodern turn' seems to offer a markedly individualistic kind of radicalism, one that feeds easily into the rhetoric of individualism where the way forward for women is lifestyle choice and self-determination largely unfettered by the erstwhile constraints of sex and gender (Skeggs 1997; Whelehan 2000). The lure of individual freedom, choice and opportunity that, on the face of it, appears liberatory might well involve opting into a putatively 'male' world of competition and self-interest that will not benefit women, or men for that matter.

Individualisation

There is a clear affinity between this projection and wider accounts of the 'individualisation' of society. Ulrich Beck and Elisabeth Beck-Gernsheim, for example, refer to 'a social impetus toward individualisation of unprecedented scale and dynamism' since the mid-twentieth century that 'forces people – for the sake of their survival – to make themselves the centre of their own life plans and conduct' (2002: 31). Women's lives, they argue, have experienced 'an individualization boost' as they have shifted from 'living for others' towards having 'a little bit of their own' (ibid.: 55). The shift in emphasis from a producer to a consumer society has entailed wide-scale social and economic change notably in the spheres of work and the family (see discussion in Chapter 6). The subjective sense of class and injustice that was crucial to class formation during industrialisation had begun to disappear from discussions of social class by the late twentieth century, to be replaced by a concern with consumption cleavages (Pakulski and Waters 1996; Savage 2000).

Consumption is at heart an individual phenomenon. As Zygmut Bauman puts it:

> Having dismantled the 'pre-modern' – traditional, ascriptive mechanisms of social placement, which left to men and women only the relatively straightforward task of 'sticking to one's own kind', of living up to (but not above) the standards attached to the 'social category' to which they were born – modernity charged the individual with the task of 'self-construction': building up one's own social identity if not fully from scratch, at least from its foundation up.
>
> (Bauman 1998: 27)

Accounts of the individualisation of society such as Anthony Giddens' discussion in *Modernity and Self Identity* (1991) stress the emergence of the self as a reflexive product. It is argued that under conditions of 'high' or 'late' modernity individuals have been released from the constraints of class and gender. Personal life has become an increasingly 'open project', an everyday social experiment that we are all more or less obliged to engage in. In terms similar to Beck and Beck-Gernsheim (2002), Giddens (1992) argues that personal and family relationships are now subject to renegotiation. This is characterised as the 'transformation of intimacy'. He claims that we are witnessing the emergence of the 'pure relationship'; no longer bound by traditional expectations of a marriage for life, we now enter into relationships for their own sake, 'for what can be derived by each person from a sustained association with another; and which is continued only in so far as it a thought by both parties to deliver enough satisfaction for each individual to stay with it' (ibid.: 58). Interestingly, Giddens positions women as the vanguard: 'women have prepared the way for an expansion of intimacy in their role as the emotional revolutionaries of intimacy' (ibid.: 130). This implies that, by virtue of a long history of expectations of nurturance, caring and greater emotional openness, women are better fitted to the conditions of life in 'late modernity' than men whose traditional identity is severely under threat.

This accords with wider popular accounts. Susan Faludi (1999), for example, refers to a 'manhood under siege'. Even though men may cling to traditional expectations of masculinity, Faludi argues that they have lost their compass in the world. Contrary to popular opinion, this is not because they have been battered by feminists' demands for change – although men very well may view it in this way (Badinter 2006; Pope *et al.* 2000). Rather, if there is a villain in the piece it is the wide-scale economic and social change, such as economic insecurity, outlined by Giddens, Beck and others, which has left men bereft of their traditional breadwinner role and emotionally unequipped to deal with the changes they face. The picture before us, even as vaguely sketched here, is one of men and women, masculinity and femininity in flux. Changes in employment such as the decline in industry and manufacturing and the increase in service sector employment, the de-traditionalisation of the family, and the rise of consumption as the basis of self (discussed in more detail in Chapters 6 and 7) all seem to contribute to the more fluid gender-based identities favoured by postmodern feminism.

But life in 'late modern' society is far from an easy ride. As Scott Lash relates, individuals have become combinards. Lacking the time and critical space for the necessary reflection to construct linear and narrative biographies, we put together networks, construct alliances, make deals. Consequently we live 'in an atmosphere of risk in which knowledge and life-chances are precarious' (Lash 2002: ix) and where the capacity for self-assertion is limited (Bauman 2001, 2002). Individualism becomes a fate, rather than a choice freely entered into. The very restlessness associated by Lash (2002) with the inability to construct linear narrative biographies is part of the market tendency to expose individuals to 'new temptations in order to be kept in a constantly seething, never wilting excitation and, indeed, in a state of suspicion and disaffection' (Bauman 1998: 26). We find an ever increasing gap between individuality as fate and individuality as practical capacity for self-assertion. Perhaps, as Bauman considers, the answer lies in standing shoulder to shoulder and marching in step, that is, condensing the individual powers of reflexivity into a collective stand and action? But this is unlikely to work. As the wealth of confessional-style television chat shows attest, the troubles that we face certainly seem to be suffered in common, but they are not additive; they simply do not add up to a 'common cause' or a totality greater than the sum of its parts. The most important similarity in our troubles lies in their being handled by each sufferer on his or her own. What we gain from the company of others is not only the resolve to confront our own personal problems alone but the worrying sense that we are in many ways responsible for our own fate.

Concepts of health

This has been very apparent in conceptualisations of health and illness. Health and illness are morally inflected (Blaxter 2004; Lupton 2003). As Ann Oakley explains, 'the body's surface is so important a marker of the individual's moral condition' (2007: 65). Jocelyn Cornwell's (1984) now classic interview study of Londoners, for example, revealed that being healthy is so intimately bound up with personal reputations – expressed in the ability to work – that people go to great lengths to present themselves as 'well', often in the face strong evidence to the contrary. This is now overlain with a new emphasis, the responsibility not only to *present* oneself as well but also to *keep* – even make – oneself well and justify illness, as staying healthy is increasingly 'politicised as a matter of personal choice and responsibility' (James and Hockey 2007: 77). Deborah Lupton cites an interview with singer Olivia Newton-John who, when accounting for her diagnosis of breast cancer, remarked, 'initially, I was puzzled that this had happened to me, because I eat sensibly, exercise regularly, don't smoke and hardly ever drink. My stress level was really high, though, so perhaps that's why this occurred' (Olivar, interview with Newton-John, cited in Lupton 2003: 100).

The individualisation that marks contemporary social life generally, and the experience of health and illness specifically, resonates strongly with the vision of both sex and gender precisely *as* malleable entities. Postmodern feminism could therefore be said to appropriately reflect the contemporary social world in which men and women live out their lives. The problem, of course, is that feminism should be critically evaluating rather than endorsing such a vision, for it not only fails to fully appreciate the profound difficulties that women face on a day-to-day basis, it seems to offer them little way out. They are caught up in identity politics that often seem far from self-evidently liberating. As Oakley puts it:

> bodies are forms and products of capitalist industry, shaped by a process that's alienating at its very core. This is the fetishism of the unblemished, youthful self. Deodorised and sexualised bodily shapes are characters in a capitalist play of commercialised symbolic meanings.
>
> (2007: 66).

This is part and parcel of the wider 'body project' of late modernity – the sense, especially among, but not confined to, the young, that the body can be made and re-made to conform to different expectations and self-expressions. The placing of health and lifestyle change high on the political and cultural agenda deflects attention from the wider political economy of health (Williams 2003) and cultivates all number of 'body hatreds', especially among women (Frost 2001).

Conclusion: treasure trove or Pandora's box?

Although feminists have worked tirelessly with and against the sex/gender distinction, it often seems to have become more a hindrance and than a help, perhaps, then, less a treasure trove and more a Pandora's box. At the present time we seem to be faced, on the one hand, with gender-specific medicine that focuses on 'given' difference and bores down to 'bits' of the biological body and, on the other, with postmodern and cultural feminism that stresses malleability and rests its gaze on the surface. Left out of the frame is any sense of the embodied or lived experience of health and illness (Bordo 1900; Davis 2007a; Klein 1996; Kuhlmann and Babitsch 2002).

Feminism is caught on the horns of a dilemma. Neither the emphasis on sex or gender 'difference' nor sex and/or gender 'diversity' seem to work unequivocally in women's favour. The strengths of each position are matched by weaknesses that can be summarised as follows. The distinction between sex and gender allowed feminists to assert that biology, at least as conceived by patriarchy, is not destiny. The argument that women's negative experience, which includes their experience of the body, is a product of *social* attributions of inferiority became the basis for a very powerful critique of women's experience of ill health and of health care. But, as we have seen in earlier chapters, two interrelated problems followed in the wake of this distinction. First, biology came either to matter too much (to 'difference' or radical feminism) or to matter very little at all (to 'equality' or liberal feminism). The second – related – problem has been the tendency to draw firm distinctions between male and female experience, be this in biological or social terms. The conceptual blinkers that arise from this are quite problematic: a built-in search for difference in the kinds of questions that we ask and, equally, those that we leave unasked. When our vision of health is so strongly coloured by fixed expectations of what specific factors – social or biological – make women ill and make men ill, then all we are likely to find is that difference.

The critical insight that postmodern feminism brings is that dichotomous thinking buys into the very patriarchal structure that feminists are trying to escape from. Since binary thinking is inherently patriarchal, the aim should be to break its stronghold rather than to sustain it. While on the face of it, (social) gender is treated as a variable, in reality it lapses back onto (fixed) binary biological difference that privileges the male body.

Here, the only effective challenge to this privilege is to appreciate *both* sex *and* gender as socially scripted. This involves doing away with (or trying to do away with) the sex/gender distinction. Patriarchy loses its moorings when experience can no longer be tied to binary difference since there is no longer an easy way to link one group (men) to all that is positive and another group (women) to all that is negative. Yet malleable identities of sex/gender not only seem to leave women without an obvious point of resistance, they are themselves bound up with the individualisation of social life (Scambler 1998). Might it be better, therefore, to view the deconstruction of sex/gender as an integral part of wider social change, rather than as a critical commentary on it? It is to this question that we turn in Chapter 6.

6   The making of women's health
Diversity and difference

It is common enough to refer to the importance of developing theory 'through the body' (e.g. Braidotti 2002; Butler 2004; Grosz 1994), but the body in question is rarely anchored in matters of life and death. As noted in the introduction to this book, where health issues are considered, interest tends to turn to reproduction, or those matters that concern body image, such as weight and eating disorders (e.g. Aapola *et al.* 2005; Brook 1999; Frost 2001; Howson 2005; Whelehan 2000). These are important, of course, but here is a general failure to go beyond this to the experience of the material body as a whole in health and illness in a changing societal landscape. As Anne Fausto-Sterling writes, 'our bodies physically imbibe our culture' (2005: 1495). In this chapter I argue that women's lives have become entangled in a social and political economy that offers them seemingly endless liberatory possibilities, but actually positions them in complex and contradictory ways with significant implications for their health, as witnessed in the shifts in life expectancies and major causes of morbidity and mortality that will be discussed in Chapter 7.

The changing landscapes of women's lives

The chapter sets out a conceptual framework for the analysis of women's health within what I will term the 'new single system' of patriarchal capitalism, a concept I introduced briefly in an earlier publication (Annandale 2003). The chapter begins by discussing the transition from the bi-polar social script of the 'old' single system to a 'new' single system wherein binary difference has not been replaced by diversity, but where both are in play and feed off each other. A review of social changes in women's lives since the last quarter of the twentieth century, taking Britain as an exemplar, shows that we should be thinking not in terms of a 'convergence' in the lives of men and women but rather of new patterns of equality and inequality. I draw upon recent thinking within materialist feminism, particularly the work of Teresa Ebert and Rosemary Hennessy, to argue that the fragmentation of the traditional bi-polar script in recent years is best conceived as the systematic effect of a new social economy that profits from the 'undecideability' of gender.

We have seen in previous chapters that the health of women and men is formed within configurations of patriarchy that vary across time and place. In this chapter I introduce the importance of the interrelationship between patriarchy and particular capitalist forms to the argument. This denotes that, where matters of life and death are concerned, patriarchy and capitalism should be understood as 'so interwoven as to be one system' (Marshall 1994: 84). The notion of a shift from an 'old' to a 'new' single system of patriarchal capitalism is used to depict and explore this process. While historically situated, these concepts are ideal types in the Weberian sense of being conceptual tools that bring together the most significant, or value-relevant, aspects of a phenomenon but that are not meant to correspond to all aspects of a specific society (Weber 1949). That is, they are used as a broad theoretical optic.

The notion of a 'single system' of patriarchy and capitalism stems back, of course, to the 1970s and 1980s, when feminists debated the vexed issue of the subsumption of gender under the economic relations of capital and labour in Marxism (referred to in Chapter 2). This laid the foundations for 'more than a decade of debate around the relative priority of capital versus patriarchy and class versus gender' within feminism (Marshall 1994: 76). So-called 'dual systems' theorists sought to identify the separate but intersecting operation of patriarchy and capital. For example, in the context of morbidity, research tends to find that when men and women occupy the same socio-economic position (something that is in itself is difficult to determine), women's health often seems to be worse than that of men. This raises the question of whether there is an 'added' or 'separate' effect of patriarchy over capitalism, or gender over class . So-called 'unified systems theory' (Young 1981) rejected attempts to determine the separate effects of capitalism and patriarchy and argued instead that capitalism is founded upon gender hierarchy. As Marysia Zalewski wrote in the early 1990s, 'the realities of patriarchy and capitalism mesh together to create a society in which men as well as women suffer oppression, but women suffer double oppression of both patriarchy and capitalism' (1990: 238; see also Bradley 2007). This was a precursor to the recognition that women's experience qua women cannot be separated out from their experience of socio-economic position (however this is defined). Of course, it is now argued in relation to health and more generally, that it is not only women who suffer this 'double oppression'. As will be discussed further in Chapter 7, this thesis is also increasingly applied to men who are positioned both as victims of socio-economic change *and* 'women's liberation' (see Jones 2002; Robertson 2007; Stanistreet *et al.* 2005).

The notion of a 'single system' discussed here, then, shares the premises of unified systems theory. The claim is that both sex (biology) and gender (social) (and the nature of their relationship) are intimately connected with particular forms of the operation of capitalism. The economic (e.g. the production and use of particular goods and commodities) and the cultural (the production and use of particular ideologies, including forms of patriarchy) are bound together. So as Donna Landry and Gerald MacLean (1993) explain, the economic and the cultural cannot be separated; the production of ideology is a material action with material effects. Table 6.1 compares the 'old' and 'new' single systems on three simplified dimensions. The 'old single system' operates by conflating sex and gender. As we have seen in previous chapters, binary divisions between the social and the biological made it possible to associate men with all that was valued (the social, mind, reason, action) and women with all that was generally devalued (biology, the body, emotion, passivity), with negative consequences to their health. Feminists sought to challenge this by slicing through the connection between sex and gender (that is, sex ≠ gender). By contrast, in the 'new single system', the bi-polar script has been replaced by greater fluidity as sex and gender both become multiple in form. As discussed in Chapter 5, the response of many feminists (and others) has been to draw attention to what (appear to be) the liberatory (or potentially liberatory) features of this fragmentation.

The 'old single system'

The notion of a bi-polar social script was first referred to in Chapter 2 where it was argued that the industrial capitalism of the early post-Second World War decades relied upon a relatively fixed and seemingly natural binary difference between men and women, built on biology. The ideology of separate spheres – which originated in the late eighteenth and early nineteenth centuries and became highly influential in defining the relations between men and women, first in the middle and later in the working classes (although, for the latter, this ideal could never actually be met) (Monahan Lang and Risman 2006; Zweiniger-Bargielowska 2001b) –

Table 6.1 Sex and gender in the 'old' and 'new' single systems of patriarchal capitalism

	Relationship between sex and gender	*Operation of capitalism*	*Feminist position*
'Old single system'	Sex = gender	Bi-polar script Binary difference relatively fixed	Sex ≠ gender
↓	↓	↓	↓
'New single system'	Sex and gender Multiple forms	Greater fluidity	Difference/ fragmentation

maintained a strong grip on experience well into the 1970s (Bradley 2007; Davidoff 1995). It grew from the earlier separation of the homestead from the workplace and work time from consumption time (Fuat Firat 1994) and was buttressed by the separation of women from much of the political and economic spheres of society (Crompton 2006a). As Donald Lowe (1995) puts it, male/female binaries were circumscribed by the industrial-capitalist system of production and social reproduction. As categories of gender were crafted onto the roles attributed to the public and private domains, sex and gender became inseparable:

> sex defined the biological qualities, but gender afforded them their meanings, roles and statuses – in short, their culture. Feminine (female) was the consumer, in the home, the private domain. Masculine (male) was producer, in the workplace, the office, the political area, the public domain.
>
> (Fuat Firat 1994: 208–9)

The bi-polar male/female distinction was a metanarrative which spilled over into most spheres of life, as depicted in Table 6.2.

Although such ideologies should not be seen as hegemonic (see discussion in Chapter 2), they were important because they provided a social order and determined the 'proper' places and positions for men and women, which were 'to support the ideals of a modern family system, which, in turn, supported a certain economic system and social formation' (Fuat Firat 1994: 209). The domestication of women was heavily influenced by the new consumer culture of the post-war period. 'The focus of 1950s life, in advertisements at least, was the family in which roles were clearly defined and in which divergences from the norm were almost unknown' (Dickason 2000: 44). The woman's job was to run the home, to care for her husband and children, and to make purchases with an eye for value for money. The man, by contrast, was largely free of such responsibilities; his job was to be the breadwinner. Thus in television product advertising the only home-based work that he was seen doing was occasional DIY, gardening, or presiding over the dinner table. 'The feminine that was signified as the consumer became the consumed, commodified, and objectified to be used

Table 6.2 The bi-polar social script

Males	*Females*
Producer	Consumer
Reasoned	Emotional/caring
Employment-oriented	Home-oriented
Active	Passive
Producers of health (e.g. physicians)	Patients (i.e. patient/waiting people)

by men' (Fuat Firat 1994: 212). Although, paradoxically, women were incited to consume, as a feminine act itself, consumption was deemed a 'passive moment, and one that required little use of reason or use of the mind' (hence the need to steer women in the right direction, discussed in Chapter 2). A man who subscribed too much, or even at all, to consumption activities risked attracting degrading labels such as 'effeminate' (ibid.: 214). 'Type A man' – competitive and hard driving – was the epitome of the bi-polar script, even though ultimately his 'coronary prone personality' was a threat to the stability of the nuclear family (Riska 2002).

The splintering of the bi-polar script

Iris Marion Young remarks that in the early twenty-first century, 'in many places the lives and spaces of women and men have become less separate, and women fill roles and appear in places that might have surprised my grandmother' (2005: 3). This change is part of the wider social tumults of recent decades. John Urry maintains that 'it increasingly seems that we are living through some extraordinary times involving massive changes to the very fabric of normal economic, political and social life' (2003: 1). He relates that, 'relations across the world are complex, rich and non-linear' (ibid.: 138) with no clear equilibrium. Although capitalism has become much more decentred with its global reach, this does not imply that its grip has weakened. On the contrary, it has become more powerful and anarchic as national controls have lessened (Touraine 1998). However, under global information and communication flows, the 'structure' of society has progressively less purchase, having given way to greater reflexivity on the part of individuals as social relations are made and remade rather than given. Social class, once the bedrock of sociological analysis, has been dubbed a 'zombie category' by Ulrich Beck (2002), actually dead for some time, but revived and inappropriately kept alive – if barely – within sociology. This does not mean that inequalities between people are diminishing – indeed, they may be hardening – but rather that they can no longer easily be understood in class – that is, collective – terms. To paraphrase Beck and Beck-Gernsheim (2002: xxiv), in the past, if you knew a man was an apprentice in a car manufacturing company, then you more or less also knew what he earned, his opinions and how he talked, the way he dressed and what he did in his spare time. The general argument is that such connections of group and grid have been swept away by the growing individualism that has accompanied the wide-scale economic changes since the last quarter of the twentieth century, with women often positioned as the vanguard.

The decline in manufacturing and rise of a knowledge economy has been accompanied by more part-time, temporary and flexible labour, more self-employment, chronic underemployment and workless households. As Richard Sennett discusses in *The Culture of the New Capitalism*, places

of employment are shifting from 'being dense, often rigid, pyramidal bureau-
cracies to more flexible networks in a constant state of inner revision'
(2006: 176). Such changes are profoundly affected by neo-liberal economic
and political ideas that have encouraged competition and promoted de-
regulation (Crompton 2006a). Zygmut Bauman depicts this process as a
shift from a 'heavy' or 'solid' to a 'light' or 'liquefied' modernity. It is
a world of more freedom, but also of radical uncertainty, a world of 'ever-
deepening wealth-and-income gaps between the better off and the worst
off sections of the world population, and inside every single society' (2001:
114). Much has been made of this in recent work on socio-economic
inequalities in health. Michael Marmot (2005), for example, argues that
differences in health do not just concern the 'haves' and 'have nots', important though this is, but rather the social processes that generate health
inequalities operate right across the social scale, top to bottom in a fine
grain. But what does this mean for women? Feminist post-colonial theory,
such as the work of Gayatri Chakravorty Spivak (2006) has been particularly
important in drawing our attention from the societal to the global level,
pointing to the essentialising of 'third world' women by framing them as
a homogenous group. The global realignments and fluidity of capital
therefore raise important questions about the kinds of racialised and
gendered selves that are produced both nationally and internationally
(Alexander and Mohanty 1997).

In the Introduction to this book, I remarked myself that we are living
through a period of striking gender-related social change in the West.
Generally, then, we can concur with Iris Marion Young that significant
change is afoot. Increases in 'human capital' – particularly in education
and work experience – has made women major beneficiaries of the new
'knowledge economy' that has accompanied the decline in manufacturing
and emergence of service industries and 'people work' (Lindsay 2003;
ONS (Office for National Statistics) 2007; Walby 2007). Taking Britain
as an example, in the mid-1970s, girls and boys left school with more or
less the same educational qualifications; thirty years later girls' achievements
were significantly outstripping boys' (Arnot *et al.* 1999). Between 1974/75
and 2005, employment levels rose from six to seven out of ten women
and declined from around nine to eight out of ten men. There have been
dramatic shifts in the kinds of jobs that men and women do. The percentage
of women in professional occupations, for example, rose from around 10
per cent in the 1970s to 42 per cent by 2005 (EOC (Equal Opportunities
Commission) 2006). In Britain, and a number of other European countries
(though not all), this has been aided by the greater facility – compared to
thirty years ago – to combine work and caring due to flexible working,
working time regulation (such as maternity leave), higher personal income
and fairer labour markets with less discrimination (e.g. equal treatment
legislation) (Monahan Lang and Risman 2006; Walby 2007: 40).

Although these contours of change suggest the popularly conceived 'convergence' in men's and women's lives, the more detailed picture is one of persisting segregation. For example, 71 per cent of British students taking A level/Higher level (high school final year) examinations in English literature in 2005 were female and 76 per cent of those taking physics were male. Although there was little difference in the percentages of women (17 per cent) and men (19 per cent) who held university degrees or equivalent in 2005, women undergraduates predominated in areas such as education and law, men in computer science and engineering. In the same year, fully 79 per cent of those working in the health and social work sector were women, and 75 per cent of those in manufacturing were men. Although segregation does not necessarily equate with better opportunities for men and worse opportunities for women, despite women's significant advancement into the higher echelons of managerial and professional jobs and an overall reduction in the 'income gap' over the last twenty years, from 29 per cent in 1975 to 17 per cent in 2005, men still on average earn significantly more than women in Britain (this is most marked in retirement where women receive 47 per cent less in weekly income than men). Moreover, part-time work attracts lower pay than full-time work, and women are far more likely than men to work part-time (42 per cent of women and 9 per cent of men worked part-time in 2005). One-third of working mothers and only one-fifth of working fathers used some kind of flexible working arrangement in 2005 (the statistics cited above are drawn from EOC 2006 and Skelton *et al.* 2007).

There is evidence of attitudinal change towards greater equality in household labour in many western societies, particularly among younger couples. For example, while in 1989 around a third of British men and a quarter of women endorsed the stereotyped view that 'a man's job is to earn money, a woman's job is to look after the home and family', in 2002 only a fifth of men and one in seven women did so (Crompton 2006b). These changes have been accompanied by a declining number of births (the total fertility rate fell from 2.95 during the 'baby boom' of the 1960s to 1.79 in 2005), later age at the birth of a first child (from the early twenties in the 1980s to the late twenties by the end of the century), a rise in one-parent households (the proportion of children in one-parent households tripled from 2 per cent in 1972 to 7 per cent in 2006), a rise in lone households (from 9 per cent 1971 to 27 per cent in 2006) and an increase in divorce (ONS 2007). As Molly Monahan Lang and Barbara Risman put it, 'as families change, so does gender. And as gender changes, so do families' (2006: 287). In Britain and elsewhere, there has been an increasing assortment and acceptability of different family forms over the last thirty or so years. Even so, broadly speaking, motherhood still involves caring and fatherhood providing, despite a general trend towards greater male involvement in child care and housework than in the past (Charles 2002; Monahan Lang and Risman 2006; Pilcher 1999). Rates of intimate partner violence (such as sexual assault, domestic violence and stalking) have been declining in Britain since the mid-1990s, but it remains the case that women are still much more likely to experience this form of violence than men (see, for example, Finney 2006). Unsurprisingly, therefore, most women's experience of heterosexual relationships is, as Lynn Jamieson (1999) discusses, some distance from Giddens' (1992) notion of the 'pure' or democratic relationship. Moreover, the wider changes highlighted are, to a significant degree, class and age-distributed. For example, an analysis of England's 2006 Key Stage 2 results (for age eleven) from the Equal Opportunities Commission (EOC) (now the Equality and Human Rights Commission) makes it clear that while on the whole girls do better, disadvantaged girls still trail behind their wealthier male peers (Skelton *et al.* 2007).

The potential of intertwined changes in education, employment, income, family formation, household structure, leisure activities and attitudes to cast long shadows over future health means that the experiences of age cohorts of women are especially important. On the one hand, there are many younger women, high in human capital, whose lives are converging somewhat with men; on the other hand, there are older women whose adult lives were built during the relatively fixed binary differences of the early- to mid-twentieth century (Walby 1997). And, of course, biological age is not the only important aspect here: age intersects with other factors that bear on life circumstances and upon health, such as social class and ethnicity. As Madeline Arnot and colleagues discuss in relation to education, girls are often positioned as ' "setting the pace of change", showing a desire for autonomy, self-fulfilment in work and family, and a valuing of risk, excitement and change', that is, a 'deepening attachment to the values of individualism', but this is highly variable (1999: 106). So despite the dramatic unfixing of young women from traditional 'gender positions' since the early 1980s (McRobbie 2000), discussed later in the chapter and in Chapter 7, for many (though not all), higher aspirations and more credentials translate into neither labour market success nor egalitarian partnerships and marriages (Delamont 2003; Hughes 2002; Walkerdine *et al.* 2001).

In the words of Sara Delamont, 'a consistent *motif* in much of the social science of the past fifteen years is that women's expectations and behaviours have changed while those of men have not' (2001: 3–4). Harriet Bradley, for example, remarks that the so-called 'gender quake' has had little impact on men; 'women's family roles and behaviors are changing, but male ideas lag behind' (2007: 129). So, as many commentators are concerned to convey, while their lives may have changed, this does not mean, as the dominant discourse would have it, that women have 'made it' (Hughes 2002). Indeed, as Christina Hughes (2002) discusses, statistical accounting of the kind undertaken above is a limited framework within which to assess the reality of changes in women's lives. Her argument that 'statistics are themselves discourses that shape responses to reality' (ibid.: 34) is well taken. The 'moral panic' about the underachievement of boys in the school system that periodically erupts at the annual reporting of school examination results in Britain and elsewhere in the world, such as Australia, is an illustration of this (see Arnot *et al.* 1999). Commentators look to the statistics to frame a particular narrative, in this case that boys are 'failing', and not that girls are 'achieving'. There is therefore always a need to look 'beyond' the statistics rather than to assume that they tell a 'given' story. In this respect, comparisons on where women stand vis-à-vis men of the kind entered into above privilege a certain kind of discourse of success that takes up the liberal feminist agenda of equality (see Chapter 3) (Hughes 2002). As now will be discussed, this is not the only, or necessarily the most useful, way to understand the relationship between women's circumstances and their health.

Changing patterns of morbidity and mortality and the experience of health and health care are taking root and growing within a social order where the old shackles of the bi-polar script have been, if not torn asunder, then decidedly worn away, to be replaced by rather more slippery silken ties. While changes in work, family, education, income and so on are an integral part of this, they can tell us only so much. The more important step is to explore how such changes have become bound up in a new social and political economy where binary difference has not so much been supplanted as combined with diversity.

The 'new single system'

Health-related oppressions – poor health, chronic illness, premature death – do not go away because women's lives become more complex and contested; they may just be different from those suffered in past times. Rosi Braidotti argues that the landscapes of what she calls late postmodernity have thrown up new subjectivities that are 'contested, multi-layered and internally contradictory'. She argues that we are witnessing the emergence of new embedded and embodied forms of 'enfleshed materialism' (2002: 13), although in common with others, she does not make any direct connections with health. It is my contention that this process can be understood through the theoretical optic of the 'new single system' of patriarchal capitalism. I develop this concept primarily by drawing on the works of Teresa Ebert and Rosemary Hennessy.

Ebert makes an important distinction between, on the one hand, what she terms 'ludic' and, on the other, 'resistance' or 'postmodern materialist feminism'. These forms share in a criticism of 'modernist' feminisms, which, it is argued, rest on a conception of 'difference-between' men and women, that is, of relatively stable binary differences, be this on biological or social grounds. They differ, however, in that, with 'ludic' postmodern feminism, the emphasis on 'difference-between' is replaced by an emphasis on 'difference-within'. Here the political project is to disrupt the 'clarity and certainty of meaning, dehierarachizing binary oppositions, inscribing the difference-within, celebrating undecideability' (Ebert 1996: 167). Ebert is critical of the work of authors such as Judith Butler (1990), Donna Haraway (1985) and Teresa de Lauretis (1987) for the weight that they place on gender as performance, for celebrating the 'play of difference' and the pleasures of 'the local, the popular, and, above all, the body (jouissance)' as the source of women's liberation (Ebert 1993: 7). She appreciates that this is a necessary move since it denaturalises dominant meanings and opens up the space for things to be different. 'In problematising politics it prevents a simple, positivistic practice and calls into questions a politics based on essentialising *differences between* seemingly self-contained and stable identities' (Ebert 1991: 293, emphasis in original). As discussed in Chapter 5, putting diversity in the place of universalising assumptions about men's and women's lives has the potential to undermine the dualities (male/female, health/unhealthy, etc.) that arise from and sustain patriarchy. However, although she does not make any reference to health, Ebert maintains that this is limited as a political strategy since it is removed from the social relations that actually *produce both* these dualities *and* their disarticulations. Indeed, as alluded to in the conclusion to Chapter 5, this kind of feminism can itself be seen as an outgrowth of the 'new single system'.

Similarly, Rosemary Hennessy recognises the value of deconstruction, remarking that it 'helps to make visible that the "real" is not given or unalterable'; however, she is concerned that much of it merely celebrates 'a fragmented, dispersed and textualised subject' (1993: 5). As she continues, 'by refiguring the self as a permeable and fragmented subjectivity but then stopping there, some postmodern discourses contribute to the formation of a subject more adequate to a globally-dispersed ... multinational consumer culture which relies upon increasingly atomized social relations' (ibid.: 6). Ebert maintains that the 'reification of highly individualistic libertarianism', including the 'privileging the erotic pleasures ("beauty")' and consumption (commodification) of the sexed/sexual body' (1996: 268), 'excludes any understanding, or even awareness, of the way women's bodies and unconscious are historically produced and exploited by the social relations of production', including the experience of millions of women worldwide who do not have such luxuries, but are 'forced by economic necessity to rent their uteruses and sell their eggs, their kidneys, and other body parts to feed themselves and their children' (ibid.: 271).

If feminism cannot, as Hennessy puts it, stop at the point of deconstruction, where does it need to go? For Ebert (1993), differences exist *in relation to* new forms of patriarchal capitalism. Undecideability itself is built into new sites of exploitation that actually rely upon a deconstruction of binary difference (again, be this on social and/or biological terms) as part of a wider critical reflexivity of the kind highlighted by Ulrich Beck, John Urry and others. As we will see later in the chapter, this reflexivity directly implicates the body and so-called health-related behaviours. Ebert asserts the need for a notion of totality, 'not seen as an organic, homogenous, unified whole' but in the Habermasian sense of 'a system of relations and an overdetermined structure of difference', where a system is always 'a totality in process, a self-divided, multiple arena of struggle' (1993: 21). Although she phrases it quite differently and in a less overtly political form, Harriet Bradley reaches the similar conclusion that 'curious though it may seem, despite complexity and diversity, societies do work and the parts of the whole do, somehow, fit together'. She believes that to account for any social phenomena accurately, we must have 'some kind of holistic view of social reality' and also that it is perfectly possible to 'have an account of the social totality that is not a totalising theory' (2007: 185). On the one hand, 'a de-centred, fragmented; porous subject' (Hennessy 1993: 9) is ripe for exploitation. On the other hand, juxtapositions of difference and diversity have the potential to generate liberatory as well as oppressive life spaces. It is women's lived experience within these spaces that requires our attention in relation to their health.

Sex/gender, health and the market economy

The restructuring of the economy, notably the shift from an industrial manufacturing to a cultural economy, is underpinned by a fracturing of the demarcations of production and reproduction, work and home, the very changes that, we have seen, have contributed so much to the changes in women's lives. It is nothing new, of course, to point to the ever-expanding place that consumption has in our lives. George Ritzer has written of the 'almost dizzying proliferation of settings that allow, encourage, and even compel us to consume' goods and services, such as the 'cathedrals of consumption' (shopping malls, superstores, theme parks, electronic shopping centres, even drop-in or McDoctor-style medical centres), which appear to offer 'increasingly magical, fantastic, and enchanted settings in which to consume' even health, it would seem – but which ultimately leave us empty and decidedly disenchanted (2005: 2, 7). As Mike Featherstone relates, consumption is not an innocent act; it is part of 'the chains of inter-dependencies and networks which bind people together across the world in terms of production, consumption and also the accumulation of risks' (2007: xvii). The interpolation of 'gender and health' in consumption, however, remains relatively uncharted territory.

It has been argued that capitalism shapes biology (and the body) in its own image (Dickens 2000). The new economy makes a virtue of the mutability of the gendered (social and biological) body as it is positioned and repositioned within new consumption practices. Not only traditional 'gender roles' (the social) but also distinctions between sexed (or 'biological') bodies are diminishing through what Hennessy (2000) calls the continual tooling and retooling of the desirous body, drawing the biological (sex) and the social (gender) into a new symphysis (Annandale 2003). As Ebert relates, this is the site where 'the economic order puts patriarchy under pressure, forcing it to allow some shifting of gendered features to meet transformations in the relations of production' (1988: 36). But 'full freedom', where men or women freely take on some or all of the attributes of the other is rarely tolerated, since it undermines the allusion of 'natural difference' that must also be kept in play. As noted in the introduction to this book, there are quite heavy cultural brakes on how far women and men can stray from the 'feminine' and 'masculine' without threatening their identities. Hence, as Ebert puts it, 'individuals are permitted to occupy bigendered subject positions – to take on *limited* attributes of the other gender – only to the degree that it is specifically required by current relations of production and only so far as the primacy of the male gender is not substantially threatened' (1988: 36, emphasis in the original). It is not only women, of course, who can suffer under this 'male primacy'. The seminal work by Robert (now Raewyn) Connell (1995) on masculinities (stressing the multiple), which has been taken up by many men's health researchers, indicates that there are 'marginalised' masculinities that suffer under the hegemonic form of patriarchy (for a recent discussion see Robertson 2007). However, given the focus of this book, it is the consequences of the continual tooling and retooling of sex and gender for women that we turn to next in this chapter.

Sex/gender isomorphism

Sex/gender isomorphism has been seized upon, indeed, advanced, by the marketing industry, as features that might once have been considered natural, such as one's sex or 'race', have acquired the 'mutability of culture' (Lury 2002). Destabilised sex/gender identities have become an indispensable condition for the cross-marketing of products and lifestyles previously identified more readily with either men or women, such as cigarettes, alcohol, and cosmetic surgery, with dubious or nebulous benefits to health and well-being. Contemporary 'self-culture' is an extremely fertile ground for the commodification of sex and gender as malleable entities. As Susan Bordo (1999) and others have discussed at some length, ' "I'm just doing it for me" has become the mantra in response to any suggestion that a person might be contemplating something like cosmetic surgery, a weight loss programme, or even just an image make-over in order to conform to someone else's – particularly a man's – ideal. It is hardly surprising, therefore, that the body in sickness and in health can be construed as one more personal project and where actions taken in its name can always be redeemed and damages reversed. As Bauman relates, since bodily life is the only life there is, 'it is impossible to conceive of an object more precious and more worthy of care' (2001: 248). Yet, we are faced with an irredeemable contradiction and thereby an inexhaustible source of anxiety: the body is an instrument of enjoyment 'and so it must be fed the attractions the world has in store', but it is also 'the most precious of possessions', which must be defended at all costs (ibid.: 248). In relation to the female body, this tension is ripe for exploitation, and this places women's health in perpetual jeopardy.

Women (and increasingly men) are positioned in diverse and contradictory ways. A good illustration of this is the Benetton clothing company, which makes diversity its brand identity. Brand iconography reveals that in the Benetton World, 'race' is not about one's skin colour, physical characteristics and so on, but about style. Benetton depicts a world no longer shackled by 'outmoded' ideas of what is appropriate for men and women (Lury 2002). For example, the autumn 2007/08 clothing collection is fronted by a young woman and man wearing almost identical 'business suits', down to white shirt and tie, the message perhaps being that business success is for men and women alike (as long as you look the part, of course). As Kathy Davis discusses in the rather different domain of cosmetic surgery, this kind of 'equality discourse' seems to create generic individuals, men and women who are 'equally subject to the pressures and ideals of beauty' (2002b: 51) and pressures to succeed. Yet global corporations such as Benetton play cleverly on both sides of the fence – keen to profit from the fissures between sex and gender (sex ≠ gender) and also to deal in traditional gendered images (sex = gender).

In 2005, Benetton joined forces with corporate giant Mattel to launch the 'Barbie loves Benetton' girls' fashion range. Branded with a pink heart logo, four dolls, tagged Paris, London, New York and Stockholm Barbie, trade in traditional female stereotypes. In 2006 Barbie 'continued around the world' to Milan, Berlin, Moscow and Beijing. As Mary F. Rogers (1999) discusses in *Barbie Culture*:

> this piece of moulded plastic represents many statuses in society – female, young adult, and white person, for starters. What it represents also derives from what her plastic persona leaves out. Barbie has no husband, daughter or son; she has no boss, no teachers, no minister or rabbi or priest, no neighbours. Her world revolves around herself and her friends, including her boyfriend Ken. Barbie may thus represent the rugged individualist in a feminine mould.
>
> (Rogers 1999: 3–4)

Barbie (in)famously has morphed into many guises to include occupations that reflect 'changing times', such as 'student', 'doctor', 'corporate executive', 'astronaut' and 'animal rights volunteer' Barbie. She has also associated herself with activities that, to judge by the doll types, now occupy women as much as their jobs, such as shopping (with 'savvy shopper' and 'suburban shopper' outfits). She has also 'acquired a panoply of ethnic "friends" and analogues that have allowed her to weather the dramatic social changes in gender and race relations that arose in the course of the sixties and seventies' (Urla and Swedlund 1995: 282). By changing her image with time – but, importantly, *not* her hyper-slim body shape and size – Barbie has become the 'perfect icon of late capitalist constructions of femininity' (ibid.: 281). As the Mattel website tells us, 'Barbie is more than a doll': she is worth $3 billion at retail (Mattel 2007). The American Girl dolls, introduced in the mid-1980s by the Pleasant Company (now a subsidiary of Mattel), have a more recent provenance than Barbie, who was created in the 1950s. Aimed at the 'preteen' (seven to twelve year old) market, the flagship line is a series of eighteen-inch 'historical dolls' and the more recent 'American Girl Today' (or 'Just Like You') dolls. The recent dolls are interesting in the context of the current discussion because although their trademark feature is that they come in combinations of face mould, skin, hair and eye colour so you can pick one that is 'just like you' – for example, doll GT3H: 'light skin, blond hair, blue eyes' or doll GTH2: 'medium skin, dark brown hair, light brown eyes' – when glimpsed side by side in the American Doll Place store on Fifth Avenue in New York, they are actually eerily alike in their Stepford Wives-like quality. The product once again is 'same, but different'.

So binary difference (which includes hyper-femininity and hyper-masculinity) and 'diversity' do not simply co-exist; they necessarily feed off each other. The vicissitudes of the 'new single system' are transferred to individual consumers who are positioned as inherently erratic themselves. The epitome of this is the young female drinker who is portrayed not only as volatile but as in need of constant reminder of her unreliability. The Christmas 2004 UK campaign of the Portman Group (which represents the alcoholic drinks industry), for example, depicted women as voluble Jekyll and Hyde characters. Dubbed 'if you drink, don't do drunk', the television advertisement featured a young woman sitting at her desk in an office. In the words of the advertising copy, 'she looks like butter wouldn't melt [in her mouth], dressed as she is in her smart business suit'. But, as the advertisement continues, when the interviewer asks her what she likes to do at the weekend, we see an altogether different side, as Ms Jekyll morphs into Ms Hyde. Along with her two friends, she is seen getting very drunk and 'putting herself and others into increasingly embarrassing and risky situations . . . starting with vomiting in the nightclub toilets and ending up in the gutter holding on to one of her friends for support'. This image was captioned with the comment: '*Not* a pretty sight'.[1]

This discourse helps to consolidate drinking as a male endeavour as 'supposed sex differences are held up as "natural" and to construe women who drink (especially to excess) as subverting their normal feminine virtues' (Day *et al.* 2004: 166). As the *Observer* newspaper put it in 1999: 'if she [any woman] drinks like a man she may start to look like one' (quoted in Day *et al.* 2004: 174). As Elizabeth Ettorre discussed over a decade ago, 'there exists at some level social disapproval and rejection' of women who are seen to be involved in 'negative drinking', since they are seen to 'put their femininity and female roles in society at risk' (1997: 14–15). The picture is further confounded since women are also held up as liberated women living in an increasingly gender-neutral world and so robbing men of one of the few remaining domains of their own, the pub or bar. British media depictions of a so-called 'ladette takeover' – reflected in commentaries such as 'a generation of women are hitting the bottle harder than men, fuelling fears of a health timebomb linked to alcohol abuse' (Marsh 2004) – co-exist with images of gender neutrality such as 'there has been a convergence of male and female taste and consumption, the way women now get tattoos, like football, watch strippers, buy erotic fiction and go on lone holidays . . . while men learn to use cosmetics, do aerobics, cook and read magazines' (Benson 2000). While outwardly more sympathetic, the book and subsequent movie *Bridget Jones's Diary* paints a rather bleak picture of women who are not really sure that they want to be 'empowered', cannot cope – Bridget is frequently seen drinking and smoking – and for whom all that matters ultimately is finding a 'knight in shining armour', in this case in the form of Mr Darcy. But the most important point in all this is the potent metanarrative within these mixed messages: liberation has let women down and in the process generated a lucrative market of unstable identities and individual women who need to be shown the light.

Selling tobacco products to women currently represents the single largest product marketing opportunity in the world (Samet and Yoon 2001). Although, as noted in Chapter 1, women have used the cigarette as a weapon of challenge to traditional ideas about female behaviour, it is unlikely that smoking would have become so popular had it not been explicitly marketed as a symbol of liberation by tobacco companies in the 1920s and 1930s (Amos and Haglund 2000). The Phillip Morris Company attributed its loss of market share in the early 1990s to the failure of Virginia Slims' longstanding 'feminist slogan', 'You've come a long way, baby', to resonate with young women. Qualities associated with feminism, such as strength and control, were judged by the company still to be important to the market; it was the old collectivist 'feminist brand' that was deemed outmoded, so it was jettisoned in favour of 'aspirational' and 'self-affirming' messages such as 'I am my own secret admirer' (Toll and Ling 2005). In early 2007, competitor company R. J. Reynolds launched the new Camel No. 9 cigarette to women. The propitious No. 9 – 'on Cloud 9', 'love potion number 9', 'dressed to the 9's', '*Channel* No. 9' – in a black pack with chamfered corners and fuchsia accents, is a 'badge product' intended to appeal to design-conscious young women. J. R. Reynolds' senior marketing manager explains that the name was chosen because it had 'a lot of appeal for being premium and sophisticated' (Stebbins quoted in Elliott 2007). It is believed that an estimated $25 million to $50 million is being spent on the launch of the product (Elliott 2007). At the time of writing, Camel No. 9 it is being aggressively marketed at launch parties in bars and clubs across the US, where women are being treated to a 'girls' night out' with traditionally 'feminine pleasures' such as having their hair styled and with take-home gift bags containing make-up and jewellery. But, although women-directed brands are important, 'unisex' or 'gender-neutral' brands still command most of the market share. As Richard Sennett (2006) discusses for cultures of capitalism generally, to sell a basically standard product, you need to magnify the value of minor differences. The challenge is to make this differentiation profitable, and it is here that brand image is all.

An interesting case of this is the marketing in Sweden of snus (or snuff), a tobacco product that is inserted under the upper lip.[2] Swedish Match promotes snus as the 'healthy alternative', a claim that is currently the subject of some debate. On the one hand, levels of tobacco-specific nitro-samines (or TSNAs) are typically a lot lower in snus than in other smokeless tobacco products, but snus is still believed to be associated with increased risk of oral cancer, pancreatic cancer, gum disease and heart disease (Cancer Research UK 2007). It is being marketed in parts of the US, but it is currently banned in the UK and all European Union countries other than Sweden. Recent research on an Australian population by Coral Gartner and colleagues (2007) reported in the medical journal *The Lancet* found little difference in health-adjusted life expectancy between smokers who quit all forms of tobacco and smokers who switched to snus. The message that the authors put across is that there are therefore health gains from switching to snus rather than continuing to smoke. In other words, it can be used in 'harm reduction' or as an aid to quitting. But it needs to be borne in mind that companies such as Swedish Match and J. R. Reynolds will not be looking to 'transfer' existing cigarettes smokers to snus (why not use both?) and will be seeking to covert non-users of any kind of tobacco to the product.

Snus is of particular interest because although it was once the preserve of men, it is becoming increasingly fashionable among Swedish women. The market green light for snus has been the banning of smoking in many western countries. You do not need to go outdoors to use snus, and it is seen as less bothersome to other people than cigarette smoke. In common with many other western countries, cigarette smoking has been declining in Sweden, but snus use has increased. Although the percentages are still small, there has been a significant increase in snus use among women over the last decade; indeed, use nearly tripled from the mid-1990s to the mid-2000s. Swedish Match (2007) reports that approximately 11,000 women aged between sixteen and seventy-five used snus daily during 2003–04.[3] Women are a target group for tobacco companies, which now market the product in flavours such as cranberry, lemon, liquorice and mint, and package it in decorated coloured small boxes as well as the traditional brownish-black plastic tins or packs (Bronholm n.d).

The lives of young women have become a dominant metaphor for social change and the touchstone for social problems in many societies (McRobbie

2000), making the stakes unduly high in relation to moral panic around their health (see also Chapter 7). But women can be construed as irresponsible whatever their age and circumstances. Older age generally, and retirement in particular, has 'become an arena more fragmented and heterogeneous in its social, economic and physical expression than ever before' (Gilleard and Higgs 2000: 45). For example, persons in their mid-fifties to mid-sixties are identified as a rising market to the alcohol industry – the very age cohort of women whose health (as will be discussed in Chapter 7) appears to be suffering a downturn relative to men. Market analysts Mintel have identified 'two new types of women' behind what is dubbed the bad behaviour trend among 'thirty- to forty-somethings': on one side is a new group of women who are single or divorced, fed up because they cannot find a partner or because they have just left one and who are saying 'to hell with the whole thing and rewarding themselves with things they enjoy like alcohol and cigarettes'. On the other side are positioned married women for whom the pressures of work and home life are growing all the time as they struggle to live up to media celebrities who at least appear to have stellar careers *and* a satisfying home life (Mintel reported in *Guardian Unlimited* 2001). Women are positioned in a multiplicity of ways, but again the overall backlash message is clear: social changes that seemingly benefit women actually have let them down, and, moreover, they cannot cope.

Conclusion

This discussion suggests that women's lives are laced with contradictions (Hennessy 2000). While it would be wrong to conclude that the changes that have been discussed are wholly negative for their health, there are indications that change is far from uniformly positive. The shackles that bound women to attributes of their (biological) sex during the 'old single system' of patriarchal capitalism have been replaced with slippery silken ties that nonetheless bind. Binary difference (even hyper-accentuated differences) and diversity exist side by side in a 'late modern' neo-liberal economy that profits from chronically unstable identities. It is more appropriate, then, to say that the 'new single system' *contains* or *subsumes*, rather than *supersedes*, the 'old single system'. Its silken ties are being woven into a new social tapestry whereby (biological) sex and (social) gender depend on each other for understanding just as much as before, but where the meaning and lived experience of biological sex and of social gender, as well as the connections between them, are far more fluid. Although the shifting warp and weft of these threads varies considerably for different women and men, speaking generally, the troubles that they weave are common enough. Thus even though there is a distinct encouragement to stretch, even cut, the binary ties, there are dangers in going too far. Accordingly, Kathy Davis (2002b) writes that cosmetic surgery might be portrayed as 'gender neutral', but this secretes a lingering worry that men who want to go under the surgeon's knife are not really normal men. They are violating their 'masculinity' in their concerns about appearance in the same way that, as we saw earlier in the chapter, women violate their 'femininity' when they 'drink' (even though there is encouragement enough from the drinks industry to do so). This discussion has addressed health only in terms of 'health behaviours' since these are one of the immediate visible fronts of the working out of the 'new single system'. The question that we must now ask is 'What are the wider consequences for women's health?' Chapter 7 considers this question by reference to changes in morbidity and mortality and with reference to reproductive choice.

7 Health in transition

Introduction

Gender-related social changes in society have the potential to reach deep into the interiors of the body and change traditional health profiles. The current chapter begins by considering the reducing 'life expectancy gap' between women and men in many western countries, changing patterns in the major causes of death, namely circulatory disease and cancer, and ways that men and women assess their own health during their lifetimes. It then considers the interpretations that researchers and other commentators have made of these patterns. It is argued that the mixed patterns of change that we are observing can be situated and interpreted within the broad theoretical optic of the 'new' single system of patriarchal capitalism, introduced in Chapter 6. Since, both historically and today, the juxtapositions of binary difference and diversity discussed in Chapters 5 and 6 seem particularly marked with reference to young women, they are given specific attention in the next part of the chapter. I consider some of the rather vexed issues raised in Chapter 5 about so-called 'postfeminism' to consider the relatively recent 'new wave' political writing by young women, asking in particular whether it has the potential to unravel the rather slippery silken ties of the 'new single system' as they implicate women's health. In the final part of the chapter I return to the longstanding feminist concern with women's reproductive bodies, discussed in Chapter 5, and reflect briefly on the conflicted spaces opened up by the new genetics and new reproductive technologies.

Changes in life expectancy

The longer average life expectancy of western women compared to men now tends to be taken for granted. However, it has not always existed, and there are indications that it may not hold true for the future. Modern statistical records go back only to the mid-eighteenth century. But reconstructed data from the early seventeenth century suggest that male and female mortality differed very little in most European countries; if anything, there appears to have been a slight male advantage (Gjonça *et al.* 2005). The now familiar female advantage began towards the end of the nineteenth century and was well established by the early 1900s. The historical shift from 'male to female advantage' was associated with changes in women's circumstances. Reductions in deaths in childbirth are often referred to in explanation, but women actually were more likely to die in earlier times from the common 'killer diseases', such as tuberculosis, scarlet fever, typhus and typhoid fever. These diseases also affected men, of course, but grinding agricultural work, chronic exhaustion from maintaining the family and the anaemia and malnutrition that resulted from an unequal share of food meant that women were less resistant to infection (Gjonça *et al.* 2005; Shorter 1982). Referring specifically to England, Sheila Ryan Johansson (1996) explains that the economic marginalisation of women was particularly marked in rural areas, as paid employment in the agrarian sector declined alongside the enclosure movement and technological change and jobs got increasingly scarce. She proposes that, as women's economic value declined, families may have found it more prudent to invest in the health of males. Industrialisation and urbanisation freed many women from the damaging effects of rural life. Of course, this does not mean to say that the experience of health and illness was the same for men and women during their lives or that there were no major differences in health between rich and poor, for men and women alike. As we saw in Chapter 2, Harriet Martineau (1861) drew attention to the needless suffering for women in occupations such as needle worker (blindness, spinal disease) or governess (perpetual fever of mind and wear and tear on nerves). But it would seem that, as far as life expectancy is concerned, the problems that arose in the wake of industrialisation affected men as much as women (Gjonça *et al.* 2005).

The hundred or so years from roughly the 1880s to around the 1970s were characterised by what now appears to have been a distinct period of gradually increasing female 'longevity advantage' in much of the West. Although this evolved differently in different countries, statistics for the UK, the US, Australia and Canada can be used to illustrate this trend. Thus in England and Wales, the number of 'extra' years, on average, that a female might expect at birth to live, compared to a male, rose from around 2 years for those born in 1841, to 3.6 years for those born in 1910, to 4.4 years for those born in 1950, to a peak of 6.9 years for those born in 1969 (ONS 2007; Yuen 2005; and see Table 7.1).[1] In the US, females born in 1900 could expect to live, on average, 2 years longer than their male counterparts; this rose to 5.5 years for those born in 1950, to reach a sizeable 7.6 years for those born in 1970 (NCHS (National Center for Health Statistics) 2004). The longevity advantage grew from 3.6 years for Australian females, and from about 3 years for Canadian females who were born at the start of the twentieth century, to a projected 7.0 and 7.1

years respectively for those born in the early 1980s (AIHW (Australian Institute of Health and Welfare) 2006; Statistics Canada 2001).

To point to this 'longevity advantage' is not to claim that women (or men for that matter) were in good health during their lifetimes. During the early decades of the twentieth century many people lacked access to the health care that they needed (as is still the case today), something that was particularly the case for women. As Helen Jones discusses, 'the plight of many single women without employment and a man to support them financially at a time when there was no free health services, was dire' (Jones 2001: 94). One of the most telling accounts of this is Margery Spring Rice's study, *Working-class Wives, Their Health and Conditions* (1939), which reports on the Women's Health Enquiry of 1933. It paints a grim picture where poverty was a way of life for all but a few and where women 'instinctively or deliberately' deprived themselves for the sake of their husband and children (ibid.: 189). Poverty was not alone in causing the 'deplorably low standard of fitness and vitality' among women (ibid.: 197). Rice reports that women were almost totally unable to look after their health due to the pressing activities of their daily lives. These concerns were, of course, those taken up some decades later by researchers concerned with women's higher morbidity when compared to men. As we saw in Chapter 3, the prevailing argument for the seeming paradox that women are sicker throughout their lives, yet live longer, has been that their 'excess' ill health is associated with chronic, often painful and disabling – but, importantly, not life-threatening – mental and physical illnesses related to the social conditions of their lives, such as lack of access to resources, exclusion from well-paid and satisfying employment and the isolation, lack of autonomy and self worth associated with caring and the 'housewife' role (Bartley 2004; Verbrugge 1983).

The reducing gap

The late 1960s and early 1970s appear to have marked a historical peak, as the female longevity 'advantage' began to be chipped away during the last quarter of the twentieth century. It should be emphasised that life expectancy/projected life expectancy at birth continues to *grow* for both males and for females, but the *gap* between them has been reducing. As we can see in Table 7.1, between 1969 and 2007 the gap reduced from 6.3 to 4 years in the UK. Table 7.2 shows that many other low-mortality Anglophone and European countries have similar patterns. Table 7.3 gives statistics for 'residual life expectancy', that is, 'life left' at different ages. Here we can see that both males and females have gained over the period 1970 to 2002, and that this has occurred at each selected point in the life course (birth, age 45 and age 65). But alongside this, we see a reducing female/male gap. Thus, at all ages, the differences are higher in 1970 than in 2002. Interestingly, as the table also shows, this narrowing gap is related to larger 'male gains' at all ages. Other countries (not shown in the table) show different trends. For example, Hungary has seen an *increasing* gap between male and female life expectancy (from 7.2 years in 1980 to 8.4 years in 2002). Here both males and females have gained years, but females have gained more years than males (Gjonça *et al.* 2005). This pattern also appears to pertain to Taiwan (Lu 2007). The gap has also increased in the Russian Federation (from 11.6 years in 1980 to 13.2 years in 2002), but in this instance, both males and females have *lost* years over the period, with men losing more than women (Gjonça *et al.* 2005).

Table 7.1 UK life expectancy

	1969 (peak)	1971	1981	1991	2001	2007	Overall 'gain'
Males	68.5	69.1	70.8	73.2	75.7	77.5	9.0
Females	74.8	75.3	76.8	78.7	80.4	81.5	6.7
Gap	6.3	6.2	6.0	5.5	4.7	4.0	

Source: ONS 2007, derived from data for Figure 7.1: Expectation of life at birth: by sex, United Kingdom.

Table 7.2 The male/female life-expectancy gap in international context (life expectancy at birth)

	1980	2002
UK	6.0	4.7
US	7.4	5.4
Sweden	6.0	4.4
Finland	8.5	6.6
France	8.1	7.4
Australia (1980–82)	7.0	4.9

Sources: AIHW 2006; Gjonça *et al.* 2005: 6–16.

Table 7.3 Residual life expectancy at selected ages (England and Wales)

	At birth			Age 45			Age 65		
Year	M	F	diff.	M	F	diff.	M	F	diff.
1970	68.8	75.1	6.3	27.2	32.7	5.5	12.0	16.0	4.0
1980	70.4	76.6	6.2	28.3	33.7	5.4	12.8	16.8	4.0
1990	73.1	78.6	5.5	30.4	35.2	4.8	14.1	17.9	3.8
2002	76.2	80.7	4.5	33.2	37.0	3.8	16.3	19.2	2.9
Gains over period	7.4	5.6		6.0	4.3		4.3	3.2	

Source: Yuen 2005: Table 1.15.

Even though intuitively we would have expected the transition to have been more traumatic for women, given threats to formerly full employment, generally speaking the massive changes in Eastern Europe following the revolutions of the late 1980s and early 1990s have negatively impacted more on the health of men than that of women (Chenet 2000). As a number of researchers have discussed, the rise in alcohol use, particularly among 'blue collar' young men, has had a lethal effect on longevity (see, for example, Cockerham 2000; Payne 2006). These international comparisons are instructive because they draw our attention to the extreme sensitivity of health status to social change, often over a relatively short period, and to the variable impacts of such change on men and women and on different age and socio-economic groups. Returning to low-mortality Anglophone and European countries, generally speaking the 'reducing gap' in mortality has resulted from accelerated improvements in longevity among males, particularly in recent years. For example, the life expectancy of western European men as a whole increased by 6.5 per cent, while that of women increased by 3.5 per cent between 1980 and 2001 (White and Cash 2004). Data from fourteen European countries show that life expectancy at birth rose on average by three months a year for men, compared to two months a year for women, between 1995 and 2003 (EHEMU (European Health Expectancy Monitoring Unit) 2005).

Although age-standardised death rates fell by about half for men and women in England and Wales between 1950 and 2004, there were significant differences in the timing of changes. Between 1950 and 1969, death rates for males under the age of seventy-five fell by 7 per cent and for their female counterparts by 23 per cent. But in the period since then, male rates have fallen by 53 per cent and female rates by 45 per cent (Baker *et al.* 2006). Most of the improvement for men has come after 1980 (Lindsay 2003). Similarly data for Canada show that the age-standardised death rate declined by twice as much for males (8 per cent) as for females (4 per cent) between 1990 and 1997 (Statistics Canada 2001). Although these changes may seem small, they are highly significant historically, since some suggest that they may eventually culminate in the end of the female longevity advantage (e.g. Connolly 2002). Generally speaking, *healthy* life expectancy falls as life expectancy increases, reflecting the burden of illness that often accompanies ageing, especially old age (ONS 2007).[2] So although on average women still live longer than men, their 'extra years' generally are not spent in good health. And as men's life expectancy increases, we might expect them to follow suit. It is interesting, therefore, to observe that research from the Netherlands has found that men's overall life expectancy not only grew more than women's between 1989 and 2000, but was accompanied by greater gains in *healthy* life expectancy (Perenboom *et al.* 2005). Bird and Rieker (2008) report a similar trend for the US. However, it is too soon to tell whether this signals a more general gap in *healthy* life expectancy favouring men. The next section of the chapter turns to changes in major causes of death to see if they to go some way towards an analysis of why the life expectancy gap is decreasing.

Major causes of death

The major causes of death in affluent western societies are circulatory disease (including heart disease and stroke) and cancer. Although men start and end with higher rates, the decrease in deaths from circulatory disease generally and cardio-vascular disease (CVD) in particular since the 1970s has been less pronounced among women than men. For example, the age-standardised death rate for circulatory disease for British men was 6,900 per million in 1971, reducing to 2,600 per million by 2005. The equivalent figures for women were 4,300 per million and 1,700 per million (ONS 2007). For coronary heart disease specifically, the decline in deaths has been slower for younger ages and, again, especially among women (Petersen *et al.* 2005).

Cancer is the second most common cause of death for British men and women. Although overall mortality rates have changed relatively little over the last thirty or so years in the UK, male deaths peaked in the mid-1980s at 2,900 per million and then fell to 2,200 per million by 2005. In contrast, female death rates peaked in the late 1980s, at 1,900 per million and then gradually fell to 1,600 per million by 2005 (ONS 2007). These overall rates conceal variations in trends for different kinds of cancer. Most notable in this respect is lung cancer. Lung cancer is far more common in men, for whom it has been the major cancer death since the 1940s. For women, breast cancer mortality was significantly higher than lung cancer mortality until it peaked in the late 1980s and lung cancer 'caught up', to the point that they are now about the same (Griffiths and Brock 2003). The timing of peaks and troughs in lung cancer incidence is quite different for British men and women. For men, both incidence and mortality rose enormously from the mid-twentieth century through to the early 1980s and thereafter began to fall, with a decrease of around 40 per cent between the mid-1970s and 2001. Incidence and mortality for women meanwhile has lagged about twenty years behind and plateaued as recently as the mid-1990s, with an increase of about 80 per cent over the same period (ONS 2006a; ONS 2007). In the US, lung cancer accounted for only 3 per cent of all female cancer deaths in 1950; by 2000 this had risen to 25 per cent (DHHS (Department of Health and Human Services) 2001).

These trends are germane to the current discussion for two reasons. First, and in simplified terms, while men are still 'worse off' than women, the incidence of these major diseases, and mortality due to them, seem to be improving at a faster pace for men than for women, thereby contributing to their overall 'catch up' in life expectancy and reduction in the 'longevity gap'. Second, CVD and many cancers are believed to be associated with so-called 'lifestyle' factors and 'lifestyle changes'. Much of the cancer burden worldwide, for example, can be attributed to the 'tobacco epidemic' (Vineis *et al.* 2004). Here the life course is important because of the cumulative effects of social circumstances in early life for later health. Age cohorts are also important, because people born around the same time are subject to similar environmental and lifestyle influences. The complex aetiology of many major diseases such as heart disease and many cancers makes it difficult to draw one-to-one associations with social factors. It also needs to be recognised that women and men appear have different biological vulnerabilities to heart disease and cancer related to underlying genetic, hormonal and metabolic differences. An illustration of this is lung cancer where there is some (as yet poorly understood) evidence that differences in gene expression increase women's risk of lung cancer at the same level of smoking (Payne 2001). Be this as it may, as Sarah Payne discusses and as has been remarked upon in previous chapters, the biological body does not exist in isolation, but develops in interaction with its social environment. Thus Payne maintains that:

> influences on both women's and men's risk of lung cancer include most obviously the fact of smoking, but this must be reconsidered in terms of what is smoked, how often, in what way and in what circumstances. Factors then affecting the impact of such smoking behaviour on lung cancer risks include responsibility for domestic work, environmental factors including cooking pollution, local pollution and environmental tobacco smoke, and industrial pollution . . .
>
> (Payne 2001: 1078)

A useful illustration of this is Taiwan, where women's rates of smoking are relatively low yet there are particularly high rates of lung cancer. In fact, lung cancer is the leading cancer death in the country for women. Between 1971 and 2001, women's age-standardised lung cancer mortality rates per 100,000 per year rose sharply from 7.83 to 14.94 (Liaw *et al.* 2005). Research by Ying-Chin Ko and colleagues (2000) pins the causal aetiology down to fumes from cooking oils, and particularly from the habit of waiting until the oil has heated to a high temperature before cooking food. Globally, this points not only to the overwhelming importance of social factors, but to the fact that the high incidence of a common disease – here lung cancer – can be related *both* to women's 'traditional' work (in the case of cooking practices in Taiwan) *and* to their 'emancipation', as discussed in the previous chapter. To add another ingredient to the pot, women and girls in Asia are currently viewed as a vast untapped market for the tobacco industry (Kaufman and Nichter 2001). If such young women are encouraged to take up smoking, it is therefore probable that both 'traditional' and 'modern' practices will put women's health in jeopardy.

Cigarettes and alcohol (again)

There is a lag effect whereby so-called health behaviours linked to the major causes of death, cancer and coronary heart disease, initiated twenty or so years earlier manifest in later life. Cigarette smoking and lung cancer is an uncommonly clear illustration of this. It has been estimated that smoking was responsible for 23 per cent of male, and 12 per cent of female deaths in the UK between 1998 and 2002 (ONS 2006a). Here we need to note that the decline in smoking has been more marked among men than among women since the last quarter of the twentieth century in many affluent western countries, and the difference in smoking prevalence has now all but disappeared in some countries (Bostock 2003; Shafey *et al.* 2003). Taking the UK as an illustration, 51 per cent of men smoked in 1974; this had fallen to about 23 per cent by 2006. For women, the drop is less evident: about 41 per cent smoked in 1974 and 21 per cent in 2006 (ONS 2008). Data for Canada show that, while 61 per cent of men smoked in 1965, only 25 per cent did so by 2001. The equivalent figures for women were 38 per cent and 21 per cent (Canadian Institute for Health Information 2003). Finally, by way of illustration, Swedish data for 2004 indicate that more women (19 per cent) than men (14 per cent) reported smoking every day (National Institute of Public Health, Sweden 2004).

The experiences of particular age cohorts are very important here. Although age patterns vary cross-nationally, the major contribution to the narrowing longevity gap in affluent societies comes from changes in adulthood. In the UK, for example, current male improvements in longevity are noticeable after the age of fifty and before the age of seventy (Gjonça *et al.* 2005). Broadly speaking, women at highest risk of lung cancer over recent years were born in the 1920s and 1930s, around the time that social impediments to women's smoking began to loosen. It should also be pointed out that smoking is a major risk factor for diseases other than lung cancer, including coronary heart disease (Unal *et al.* 2004).The cohort effect in smoking is likely to be a significant contributor to the narrowing longevity gap from around the 1970s since, by this time, women born in the 1920s would be around sixty years old and already subject to the negative effects of smoking (Waldron 1993). Male smoking rates and lung cancer deaths were already declining by this time. This trend seems unlikely to diminish in the near future given that in a number of countries many teenage girls and younger women are now more likely to smoke than boys (European Commission 2000). Moreover, research shows that the smoking epidemic within a country tends to go though stages, beginning with men in higher socio-economic status groups, followed by women in the same strata, then spreading to men, and then to women, in lower socio-economic groups. The particular timing of this process in western countries means that the burden is now increasingly borne by women in lower socio-economic groups and that it is associated with multiple disadvantage (Bostock 2003; Harman *et al.* 2006).

Alcohol consumption above daily recommended rates, and especially 'binge drinking', is indirectly associated with CHD (Unal *et al.* 2004). Despite what we might be led to believe from the moral panic over 'young women's drinking' (see Chapter 6), cross-nationally, men still consume considerably more alcohol than women (Bird and Rieker 2008; ONS 2007; Payne 2006). To take the UK as an example, in 2005, just over one-third of men and one-fifth of women reported exceeding the recommended daily amount of alcohol in 2005 (ONS 2007).[3] A total of 30 per cent of young men aged 16–24 had engaged in binge drinking (defined as at least twice the recommended daily amounts) in the week before interview, compared to 22 per cent of girls in the same age range (ONS 2007). Among men, there appears to be little variation by social class, although for women, higher levels of drinking seem to be associated with higher social class, at least as measured by occupation (ONS 2007; Waterson 2000). Recognition of this has no doubt fuelled concerns over an association between women's movement into the higher echelons of the workforce and 'bad health behaviours'. However, although males generally consume more alcohol than females, the percentage of adults consuming more than the recommend weekly level in Britain has remained more or less stable among men since the mid-1990s, but increased by over 50 per cent among women (General Household Survey cited by Petersen *et al.* 2005). By way of further illustration, although by international comparison levels of alcohol consumption are relatively low as a whole in Sweden, consumption has been rising.[4] Here, too, men still drink more than women, but there has been 'convergence between sexes, at least in urban areas' (Helmersson Bergmark 2004: 297).

Alcohol-related death rates have increased significantly in the UK and elsewhere in recent years. The UK, for example, saw a rise from 6.9 to 12.9 per 100,000 population between 1991 and 2005. However two-thirds of this increase was attributable to male deaths with the gap between males and females widening over the period (ONS 2006c). There has been a distinct rise in mortality from chronic liver disease and cirrhosis among both English men and women from the early 1990s. Although female rates remain lower than male rates, they have risen more sharply and are currently above the average of the original fifteen European Union (EU) member states (DoH (Department of Health) 2007). There is evidence that women are more biologically vulnerable to health damage from alcohol: in addition to having different body mass, men and women metabolise alcohol differently, so that women reach higher blood alcohol levels than men while consuming similar weight-adjusted amounts of alcohol (Bird and Rieker 2008; Waterson 2000).

Self-reports of health

Age at death is a relatively robust indicator and historical data enable us reliably to review trends over time. While we would expect a relationship between mortality and morbidity in terms of the major causes of death that have been discussed, this may tell us relatively little about the overall state of a person's health during their lifetime. It is very difficult to track morbidity (or illness) patterns over time, since any observed changes could reflect changing thresholds of 'what counts' as illness and changes in symptom reporting. This would be confounded by any changes in how men and women (and different subgroups of men and women) think about and act on symptoms. So data are not strictly comparable (Payne 2006). With these significant caveats in mind, at the present time at least, male/female morbidity differences in adulthood appear to be relatively small (Payne 2006). When one looks internationally and also at different studies within countries, the figures are inconsistent: in some contexts women seem to report slightly poorer health; in others there is little or no difference (Payne 2006); and in others still, men report their health to be worse. To take a specific illustration, data for self-assessed health, longstanding illness and acute sickness collected annually for England show gradual and slight increases in reports of ill health on all measures for both men and women between 1993 and 2003. At each time point, ill health inclines modestly towards women, but the overall picture is more of similarity than difference (DoH 2004). Data from Australia on self-assessed health for 1995 and 2001 also show minimal differences; if anything, there are better ratings in some age groups among women in 2001 (AIHW 2004). The picture is, of course, complicated for different age groups and for some specific conditions. For example, a much larger proportion of older women suffer from musculoskeletal conditions such as arthritis and rheumatism than men (see, for example, GHS (General Household Survey) 2004). As, discussed in Chapter 3, it is possible that a series of urban myths have formed around women's 'excess' morbidity (Macintyre *et al.* 1999) whereby researchers have been blinkered in the study of morbidity patterns by the search for difference in relation to the sex (biology)/(social) gender distinction.

Social class and ethnicity

Patterns of health and illness in contemporary western societies are highly complex and therefore defy easy summary, particularly when we bear in mind that health status is about far more than just being a woman or a man, that is, when we take into account factors such as age, ethnicity and social class. It is beyond the scope of this book to explore this in anything near the depth and detail that is required for a complete understanding. However, it is important to point out that the splintering of the bi-polar social script discussed in Chapter 6 has meant not only new patterns of equality and inequality between women and men but also new patterns of inequality between women. Thus as Sylvia Walby (1997) remarks:

to a significant extent women are polarising between those, typically younger, educated and employed, who engage in new patterns of gender relations somewhat convergent with those of men, and those, particularly disadvantaged women, typically older and less educated, who built their life trajectories around patterns of private patriarchy. These new patterns are intertwined with diversities and inequalities generated by social divisions including class, ethnicity and region.

(Walby 1997: 2)

There are limitations in using conventional statistical measures of socio-economic status to capture women's experience (Bartley 2004). However, data often show marked health differences within women (although they are often less strong than those among men). To take Britain as an example, although mortality rates have been declining, social class differences (measured by occupation) retain a strong grip. Thus for the period 1997–2001, the life expectancy of women in occupational class V (unskilled) was 77.6 years, compared to 82.2 years for women in class I (professional) (ONS n.d). Age-standardised all-cause mortality ratios of classes IV and V : I and II (per 100,000 person years) for women were 1.69 in 1986–92 and 1.41 in 1997–99 (White *et al.* 2003; for a wider discussion, see Graham 2000). Differences in health also vary by ethnicity, with many minority ethnic groups (but not all) reporting worse health than the 'general population'. For example, data for England show that, while 44 per cent of black Caribbean and 44 per cent of Irish women reported a long-standing illness in 2004, only 24 per cent of Chinese and black African women did so (Sproston and Mindell, cited in Field and Blakemore 2007).

Convergence?

The association of the narrowing 'longevity gap' with growing societal affluence explains its concentration in high-income, low-mortality Anglophone and European countries and also prompts commentators to find explanations for the trend in the changes in employment patterns, in family structures and in the apparent convergence in the 'lifestyles' of men and women that these countries have experienced.

It therefore is not surprising that a broadly conceived 'convergence thesis' has been adopted by social scientists. Thus Mel Bartley writes that:

we might guess that as the home and work situations of women and men become more similar (as women become more likely to have full-time jobs of similar status to men, and as work and marriage and children are combined in more similar ways), any remaining health differences between men and women may disappear.

(Bartley 2004: 139–40)

More generally, Ingrid Waldron dubs this the 'women's emancipation thesis', or the view that 'the changing roles of women and a general liberalisation of norms concerning women's behaviour have resulted in decreasing gender differences in mortality' (2000: 152). Others place their emphasis on changes among men. Thus Jacques Vallin and colleagues (2001: 165) refer to men cutting back on 'certain harmful habits which were previously markedly male in nature (alcohol and tobacco consumption, for instance)', whereas women are taking them up (though not to the same extent) (2001: 165). They also draw attention to factors such as reduced male exposure to risks due to safety improvements on the roads and at work, and to men 'beginning to copy women in their attitude to health', such as making more frequent use of health services (although, again, women's use generally remains higher) (ibid.: 165).

While these authors draw attention to positive change in men's lives, there is also a propensity to cast men as victims buffeted by the winds of rapid social change but also subject to the heavy drag of traditional patriarchy. There is some merit in this argument, particularly when attention is drawn to the difficulties experienced by sub-groups of men, such as young working-class men who are suffering from high levels of unemployment (McDowell 2003). But this 'crisis discourse' also harbours difficulties, because, as Stephen Whitehead relates, it polarises debate 'into one of competition for health resources between women and men, while also enflaming the "moral panic" and ensuing backlash against feminism and women's issues generally' (2002: 52–3). This is particularly evident when researchers foreground women's 'advantages' (such as longer life expectancy, greater use of health services and so on) *in order to* establish men as the disadvantaged (see, for example, Meryn 2004; White and Holmes 2006).

Even more problematic is the wider literature that castigates women for the sorrows of men as it filters into discussion of health. Harrison G. Pope and co-authors, for example, draw an association between what they see as a growing preoccupation among men of all ages with their bodies, or what they call 'the Adonis complex', and anxiety and depression. Such an association may well exist – suicide rates are, for example, much higher in males than females.[5] But the concerning point is their conclusion that the reason *why* men are left with 'primarily their bodies as the defining source of masculinity' is the 'growing equality between women and men in many aspects of life' (Pope *et al.* 2000: 48, 50). Wider support for this thesis is found in the 'backlash' literature (referred to in Chapter 5) written by men and women alike, which berates feminists for failing to acknowledge women's new advantage and for failing to appreciate the problems of men (see Coward 2000; Jones 2002). Combined with the depictions of individual women making (misguided) choices, that is, as having failed in their 'own emancipation' (discussed in Chapter 6), it is a fairly short step to the conclusion that women are liable not only for their own 'downfall' but also for that of men (and, on occasion, for society as a whole). Although my focus in this book is on women, locating both the health of men and women in the context of the 'new single system' of patriarchal capitalism may help to avoid what seems to have become a victim-blaming approach.

Conflicted spaces

It has been argued that the old shackles of the binary social script, which positioned women and men as opposites, have been superseded by a more flexible social system or, as I have put it earlier, by slippery silken ties that nonetheless bind. The new fabric of life for women is laced with contradictions (a point that applies to men too) with implications for their health. This is not to imply that things were totally clear cut in the past, but rather that the change is a matter of degree, although the scale is large. Thus we have seen that in low-mortality and Anglophone countries, women's advantage in life expectancy is being chipped away. It is ironic, to say the least, if it is the case that women were more protected by the binary divides of the 'old single system'.

As Penny Kane (1994) proposed some time ago, theoretically there are three possible explanations for the reducing male/female gap in life expectancy: it could be due to improvements for men; there could be a deterioration or plateauing for women; or both of these trends could be taking place simultaneously. The latter explanation has the greater validity. Thus, men are indeed 'catching up', but it has to be remembered alongside this that, at least on average, women's life expectancy is not *decreasing*. However, there is very clear evidence of deterioration in some causes of death, with the exponential rise in the prevalence of lung cancer and lung cancer mortality among women being the obvious example. But drawing on the arguments of Fred Pampel, this cannot in any simple or easy sense be attributed to women's 'independence'. Using data from several countries, Pampel shows that it is not so much how 'egalitarian' a country is, in terms of women's 'emancipation', that accounts for levels of smoking but where a country stands in terms of the diffusion of the smoking epidemic that seems to matter. Thus, 'the longer the history of smoking in a nation', 'the more alike the smoking of men and women is' (Pampel 2001: 400; see also Pampel 2002). There have been sharp increases in liver disease and deaths from cirrhosis of the liver among women in recent years, but it is still the case that incidence is higher among men. Heart disease is the major cause of death for both men and women, but women's rates remain lower than men's. As noted above, there are also significant differences *among* women (and among men), such as those related to social class. Moreover, people typically do not present with a neatly packaged profile of health 'risks' or 'benefits' in the ways that they live their lives (Bird and Rieker 2008). Thus, in Britain, women in poorer socio-economic circumstances tend to smoke more than their better-off counterparts, but the better off in their turn tend to be the consumers of 'excessive' amounts of alcohol.

The weft and weave of the fabric of life is finally complicated by the knotty issue of how men and women feel about the state of their own health, which, in terms of general assessments, often seems more similar than different but varies in relation to specific symptoms and conditions (Annandale and Field 2007). The way that I have discussed health has been self-evidently limited. The difficulty, of course, is that health is multi-faceted. As sociologists of health have been arguing for some time, the ways that individuals think about their health, its relationship to their identity, and how they interpret symptoms and take actions in relation to their health is complicated enough (Blaxter 2004; Herzlich 1973; James and Hockey 2007). Identifying why it is socially patterned in particular ways adds an even greater challenge, and it has been possible to touch upon only some aspects of this here.

In the place of the convergence narrative, I propose that these complex and shifting patterns of health and illness can be interpreted though the lens of the multiple positioning of women in relation to what I have called the 'new single system' of patriarchal capitalism (although it has to be appreciated that this too is a constructed narrative in its own terms). In some ways this position shares the view of Ingrid Waldron that 'recent trends in gender differences in behaviour have been influenced by the interacting effects of fundamental aspects of traditional gender roles and the contemporary context' and that this has led to a diversity of experience (2000: 154). But it differs from this by emphasising, among other things, the systematically driven nature of these complex shifts. As Wendy Brown discusses, but without reference to health, we need an approach that 'discerns structures of dominance within diffused and disorienting orders of power, thereby stretching toward a more politically potent analysis than that which our individuated and fragmented existences can generate' (1995: 51). It will be remembered from Chapter 6 that in the Weberian (Weber 1949) conceptualisation of an ideal type, the new single system is put forward as a broad theoretical optic to depict not simply the co-existence of binary difference and diversity (be this on social and/or biological grounds) but also their necessary interweaving.

Through the optic of the 'new single system' we can appreciate that the old balance of power has indeed changed; that the rigid orthodoxies of the past are breaking down and being reconfigured in new, more complex ways with implications for health, and that these changes are systematic in form. As we saw in Chapter 6, at the level of the social economy, the operation of the 'new single system' is discernible in juxtapositions of diversity and binary difference that co-exist and necessarily feed off each other. Reading social reality in this way assumes the mantle of political critique not only by widening the scope of what we see but by starting from a different place in *what* we see (Hennessy 2000). However, it is essential to also be aware that these ideologies are tapestries woven out of contrary impulses, which themselves resist a final suturing. As Teresa

Ebert writes of what she terms late capitalist patriarchy, the effect is not an organic, homogenous, unified whole, but rather an over-determined 'totality in process, a self-divided, multiple arena of social struggle' (1993: 21). Although it appears – to borrow an image from J. K. Gibson-Graham (1996: 258) – that our lives are 'dripping with' what I have termed a 'new single system' of patriarchal capitalism; that is, unitary, singular and total, juxtapositions of difference and diversity are historically specific ideological effects that generate liberatory as well as oppressive life spaces. These spaces can never be pristine and sharply bounded. Rather, they are inescapably muddied and conflicted. I conceptualise these as the 'conflicted spaces' of the 'single system' of patriarchal capitalism.

The data presented above are rather sterile, aggregated snapshots of undistinguishable individuals with particular diseases, or who died, or are projected to die, at particular ages. Genetic and biological influences notwithstanding, they inevitably mask the fundamentally dynamic nature of 'health status' as it is shaped by the circumstances of our lives. Much of what happens to us and the decisions we take in our daily lives affects our health in one way or another, although we are generally unaware of, unable or unwilling to fathom exactly how at the time (Bird and Rieker 2008). As we have seen, the eddies of the 'new single system' generate heavily conflicted milieu – spaces for those things that are beneficial and for those things that are detrimental to health (or both – cigarette smoking, for example, may help with short-term stress while undermining longer term well-being). As Stephanie Genz discusses more generally, women's use of 'different dimensions of agency' slip between 'feminised agency and patriarchal recuperation' (2006: 346). Hybridity is the reality of our lives as we 'buy into standardized femininities while also seeking to resignify their meanings' (ibid.: 338). It is our lived or embodied experience within the 'conflicted spaces' of the 'new single system' that requires our attention in relation to health.

'New Feminism'

I have noted at a number of points in the book that the anxiety that gender-related change has evoked throughout history makes the stakes unduly high in terms of moral panic around the health of young women. In Chapter 1, I quoted Charlotte Perkins Gilman who, writing at the age of seventy-three in 1923, expressed her worries about the 'new women' of the early twentieth century, whom she castigated as imitating the vices of men and as 'painted, high-heeled, powdered, cigarette-smoking idiots' (Gilman 1963 [1935]; Gilman cited in Lane 1997: 342). More recently – since the closing decades of the twentieth century – the periodic eruption of concern in the popular media about young women as 'liberated but paying the price' in relation to their health makes them a worthy focus of attention here.

In Chapter 5, I considered the recent feminist 'backlash' literature (e.g. Coward 2000; Roiphe 1993; Wolf 2006), which maintains that feminism is not only outmoded and irrelevant to the contemporary world but also partially responsible not only for the problems that women face but sometimes also for those faced by society as a whole (Oakley 1998). In distinction to this literature, there is a body of writing by 'third' or 'new wave' feminists that does not so much argue that feminism is not needed but that it needs a radical restyling. Nonetheless, this 'new generation' writing has been subject to significant criticism for its individualistic ethos and therefore of too casually claiming that 'clear victories have been won and that the way forward is in the form of lifestyle choices and self-determination' (Whelehan 2000: 11). This said, as Astrid Henry (2004) discusses in *Not My Mother's Sister*, there is perhaps a need for all feminisms to be 'peer driven' in order to be seen as relevant to their day and, most crucially, as appreciative of the circumstances of women's lives at the time.

Is there then, as Sinikka Aapola and co-authors write, evidence that some young women are developing new kinds of feminisms, feminisms that are more relevant to the socio-economic conditions of late modernity, in the manner of the oft-quoted phrase, 'I'm not a feminist, but . . .'? Or should these new ways of thinking be conceived as rejecting feminism altogether? (Aapola *et al.* 2005). And, either way, what might this mean in health terms? In their book *Manifesta*, which mainly relates to the US context, Jennifer Baumgardner and Amy Richards remark that, 'it's a sign of the times that feminists today are more likely to be individuals quietly (or not so quietly) living self-determined lives than radicals on the ramparts' (2000: 26). But they continue that this does not mean to say that they have no interest in, and do nothing about, issues such as abortion, sexually transmitted diseases (STDs), rape and violence. Feminism, they argue, has been 'expanded' to include any number of positionalities. Similarly, in the English context, Emma Rich concludes that the young women in her study were 'negotiating their lives around a gender dynamic', even though they saw feminism as a thing of the past (2005: 495). And Aapola and colleagues found that, even though young women may 'feel alienated from or express disinterest in feminist ideology, labels or politics, their identities and world views are deeply shaped by feminist frameworks' (2005: 196). Thus they conclude that young women are attuned to 'diversity and the need for feminisms grounded in multiplicity' (ibid.: 210). 'Girlhood', they remark, 'has become a receptacle for social anxieties about change', but it is also a site of new possibilities, places and modes for their feminist theory and practice' (ibid.: 216).

At the risk of over-generalisation, the defining features of 'new wave' feminism are the notions of entitlement and individualism. Angela McRobbie refers to an almost brutal individualism that 'turns all social relations into an extension of the market economy' as women's traditional identities are unhinged by consumption (2000: 211). Crucially, instead of being opposed, femininity and feminism are drawn into a new alignment. At the hybrid of the two is what has been dubbed 'free market feminism'; as Imelda Whelehan (2000) puts it, assertive and self-seeking but reliant on feminine allure. Young women buy into standardised femininities and seek to resignify their meanings (Genz 2006). As Susan Hopkins puts it in her book of the same name, there are many 'girl heroes', from the popularisers of so-called 'girl power' such as the Spice Girls to the media celebrities (such as the wives and girlfriends of premier league footballers, dubbed WAGS in the UK) to whom many girls and young women look, 'not just for entertainment but for self-definition, meaning and purpose' (Hopkins 2002: 182). Perhaps the most contentious of these resignifications is what has been called 'raunch culture' in the US and is approximated in the UK, at least in the 1990s, by the notion of the 'ladette' (referred to in Chapter 6). Ariel Levy concludes that 'raunch' is essentially commercial, trading in 'kitschy, slutty stereotypes of female sexuality' (2005: 76) filmed for reality TV spectacle. As a rebellion against traditional femininity, it is perhaps the most easy 'new feminism' to see as recuperated by the traditional masculine sexual imagination. Thus Harriet Bradley believes that 'raunch' is 'indicative of what may happen when strict boundaries established by gender roles and rules are challenged: women take on practices and behaviours defined as "masculine" and not the other way round' (2007: 165). Rather than seeing this as somehow inevitable, perhaps we should follow Beverly Skeggs' (1997) point that 'new feminisms' are themselves very marketable.

A comparison can be drawn between 'raunch culture' and the Riot Girls (or Grrrls) of the early 1990s, a loose group of punk-influenced feminists in the US. As Baumgardner and Richards discuss, the Riot Grrrls 'reclaimed and defanged epithets that kept young women in line, such as "slut" and "fuck no fat chicks", by scrawling these words on their bodies' (2000: 78; see also Hopkins 2002). They also 'reclaimed space for women' in punk rock by 'deflating the construction of the feminine' by adopting a girlie kind of dress matched with combat boots and the previously referred to slogans (Archer Mann and Huffman 2005: 71). Grrrlpower, or power feminism, influenced books, fanzines, web pages and music. By focusing 'on girls as capable, tough, articulate and reflective . . . [i]t reclaims the word "girl" and sometimes focuses on young women's anger as a feminist tool' (Aapola *et al.* 2005: 203).

This then is activism of a different kind to that discussed in Chapter 2 in relation to the women's movement of the 1960s and 1970s. To be sure there are jeopardies, such as an assertiveness that is ultimately reliant on feminine allure (Whelehan 2000), but nonetheless there is also an appeal to the argument that 'gender inequality' has become a 'collective problem with an individual solution' (Budgeon 2001: 18). A contentious illustration of this is Periel Aschenbrand's promotion of 'body as billboard'. As she puts it:

I was like, the whole point is that people are constantly staring at our tits, right? And people are constantly staring at our tits because our bodies are objectified because our tits are oversexualized, right? It follows, then, that we should take advantage of this fact, right? . . . I think we should be putting our tits to better use – it's prime advertising space being used on vapid slogans like "Princess". Instead of turning us into a bunch of apathetic morons, T-shirts should say things like . . . 'By 2020, 100 million people in Africa will have died of AIDS'.

(Aschenbrand 2005: 66).

Susan Archer Mann and Douglas Huffman neatly summarise the 'new wave' feminism as focusing 'more on the individual than society; more on internalised than external expression; and more on culture than on material life' (2005: 86). Consequently many of the 'young feminist' anthologies contain personal narratives 'about the contradictions, uncertainties, and dilemmas they face in their everyday lives' (ibid.: 70–1). An illustration of this is *Smashed, Growing up a Drunk Girl* (Zailckas 2005). In this autobiography, Koren Zailckas concludes that young women drink due to unhappiness. Thus she tells the reader that she drank to excess due to self-loathing, because she felt 'shamed, self-conscious and small' (ibid.: xiv). She is insistent that women's drinking in this way is not aping men, nor is it a manifestation of 'girl power'. Yet upon reading the book it is hard *not* to conclude that her feelings were in no small part due to living in a male-controlled and male-defined world. Thus she writes that:

the thing I am discovering about girldom is, in the end, nobody cares is you are a drunk, an anorexic, a runaway, a dropout, a dope fiend, or a psychotic. These things aren't regaled, but they are allowed. With the right amount of therapy or religion or pharmaceuticals, they can be passed off as life stages. That is, as long as you are still a virgin. To be a whore is unsalvageable.

(Zailckas 2005: 77–8)

Moving between the 'feminized agency and patriarchal recuperation' that Genz (2006: 346) and others describe is an inevitability in the 'new single system'. Moreover, as noted earlier, the strains of individualism ring loudly, as the second wave feminist notion that the 'personal is political' is reversed to become 'the political is purely personal' (Archer Mann and Huffman 2005: 74). So:

in a world where simulations increasingly blur the line between artifice and reality [. . .] it is not surprising that certain strands of third wave feminism have taken a more idealist track that loses sight of the social and material conditions that created a world where difference, decentering and deconstruction became ever more prominent.

(Archer Mann and Huffman 2005: 82)

No doubt because of their metaphorical status as harbingers of unwanted change (McRobbie 2000), most attention has been given to young women in this regard, but as Amanda Grenier and Jill Hanley discuss, older women may use feminised conceptions such as the 'little old lady' tactically, sometimes resisting classifications of their bodies in decline, at others using them to achieve certain ends (2007: 222).

This discussion highlights the highly conflicted milieu in which personal identities are constructed. It demonstrates above all the 'lived messiness' (Heywood and Drake 1997; Tong 2007) that is the fabric of women's lives within the 'new single system'. To frame this in terms of Teresa Ebert's (1993) problematic (outlined in Chapter 6), differences certainly arise – the different expressions of 'power feminism' discussed here signal this – but crucially these are *'differences-in-relation'* to the current forms of patriarchal capitalism. Thus the 'new single system' contains or subsumes the 'old single system' as binary difference and diversity co-exist side by side. A further illustration of this process will now briefly be given by reference to new reproductive technologies.

Reproductive technologies

Adele Clarke and Virginia Olesen remark that 'late capitalism has fallen in love with difference (Clarke 1995), and difference is moving into medicine – along with capital' (Clarke and Olesen 1999: 18). As these authors continue, the 'difference project' within feminism and within biomedicine 'is and will continue to be central to revisioning women, health and healing' (ibid.: 18). This is nowhere more evident than in the field of new reproductive technology. In Chapter 4, I discussed Shulamith Firestone's (1971) early argument that technology provides the opportunity to free women from their 'reproductive tyranny'. Firestone was, of course, referring specifically to the potential of technology to break the blood tie to the mother and thus 'do away with' what she saw as the false dichotomy that biology has created between men and women. The response at the time and subsequently has been highly contentious.

For some, assisted reproductive technologies (ART) such as gamete intrafallopian transfer (GIFT) and in vitro fertilisation (IVF) provide opportunities that would otherwise not have been available to them to become a parent. Similarly, prenatal screening techniques related to genetics or blood or serum collection, such as chorionic villus sampling (CVS), maternal serum screening and amniocentesis hold out the possibility of giving birth to a 'healthy' baby, which otherwise might not have been likely. ARTs also provide the opportunity to deconstruct conventional understandings of the 'efficient' and 'inefficient' female and, to some extent, also male bodies, and open up the space for new forms of parenting, which are made possible when the mother–biology–woman link is severed (Sawicki 1991). For Morag Farquhar (1996), ARTs are a challenge to familiar narratives such as who should count as a parent, a child, kin. Thus 'they invite creative rethinking of traditional identity categories and openness to new provisional and hybrid ones' (ibid.: 10). As Margrit Shildrick puts it, they 'cut across hitherto entrenched categories of difference (fertile/infertile; young/old; lesbian/heterosexual; and potentially human/animal)' (1997: 181).

Yet, for others, ARTs are highly problematic. They are a further way of disciplining female bodies as they become even more strongly marked as 'public property' (Balsamo 1996). Thus Anne Balsamo writes that 'reproductive technologies provide the means for exercising power relations on the flesh of the female body' through the authority relations of science (1996: 82). Perhaps the best-known set of arguments in this regard comes from the Feminist International Network of Resistance to Reproductive and Genetic Engineering (or FINRRAGE), which was formed in the mid-1980s, and sees gene technologies such as pre-implantation genetic diagnosis (PGD), prenatal testing and new reproductive technologies as tools of eugenic racist and sexist ideologies. As Marysia Zalewski discusses, from this vantage point, women's subject-hood is placed in jeopardy. Reproductive technologies are 'harmful to women in a number of ways – controlling them, fragmenting them, dismembering and experimenting on them' (Zalewski 2000: 78). Elizabeth Ettorre argues that with reproductive genetics, reproduction is exhibiting signs of becoming a regulatory system 'focused on the replications of bodies which must exemplify completeness (i.e. organs, limbs, torsos, crania filled with brains etc.), health, well-being, individual potential and future welfare' (2002: 3). Through this, 'an assortment of disciplinary strategies (i.e. biomedical knowledges, technologies, etc.) attends to the pregnant body to construct and normalise it' (ibid.: 3). In other words, genetics is not only a disciplinary process but also a gendered disciplinary process.

Moreover, in an age of 'transnational feminisms', there are significant divisions between women who profit from new reproductive technologies and those who are exploited by them, as made clear by Jyotsna Agnihotri Gupta's (2006) discussion of the global market in reproductive body parts and reproductive services. Thus:

> initially confined to solid organs, such as kidneys, livers and hearts, with the development and expanded use of IVF technology, the last decade of the twentieth-century saw this extended to reproductive body parts, such as sperm, ova and embryos, which have become discrete entities – commodities that can be donated or traded, by individuals themselves as well as infertility specialists, IVF brokers, etc., for profit.
>
> (Gupta 2006: 29)

Techniques such as IVF, and imaging technologies such as ultrasound, are therefore invested with multiple meanings. The combination of promises and threats (Dumit and Davis-Floyd 1998) that they hold out is unavoidable. Thus Margrit Shildrick relates that, whatever else ARTS have in common, 'all are concerned in more or less sophisticated ways with diversifying those limited things of which particular bodies are capable' (1997: 180). They can be a form of monitoring and surveillance, such as checking on the 'efficiency' of the female body, yet also productive of new subjectivities, for example, the new baby and the new mother (or father) through visualisation. Yet, as Gupta also puts it, since the 1980s there has been a shift 'from the credo "our bodies, our selves" popularised by the Boston Women's Health Book Collective in the 1970s, to "my body, my body parts"' (Gupta 2006: 33). In other words, significantly contrasting identities can be formed in relation to the use of assisted reproductive technologies.

Conclusion

In this chapter I have picked up the threads begun in Chapter 3 in relation to women's health status and their reproductive health. I argued in Chapters 3 and 4 that these two strands of work grew out of the distinction between sex (biology) and gender (social), which was initially engaged to counter the patriarchal conflation of women with their (inferior) biology. This distinction was a conceptual treasure trove for research on women's health, but one that nevertheless has harboured problems. Not the least of these was the fragmentation of research on women's health. As we have seen, research on health status has emphasised the *social* production of health and illness within a predominately liberal or equality feminist framework. The inevitable consequence of this has been a neglect of the interaction of the social and the biological and a generally reductivist approach, which overlooks the wider social relations of gender. By contrast, radical feminist inspired research on reproductive health and childbirth brought reproduction right to the heart of feminism. The problem, however, was that, more often than not, the focus was upon biological difference.

By the 1980s it was becoming clear that the focus on difference, be this on social and/or biological grounds, was an inadequate basis for the analysis of women's lives and their health in an environment where their experiences were increasingly marked by diversity. Many social scientists, feminists included, began to argue that a theory built on distinction is of little relevance in a complex world of fast-paced change and where both the social (or gendered) and the biological (or sexed) body is modifiable and no longer annexed in any simple one-to-one way with either women or men. I have argued, however, that binary differences have not so much been supplanted as combined with diversity in a world in which the social and the biological are drawn into a new, shifting and even sometimes more pernicious relationship than in the old binary social script. This new relationship has been conceptualised as a 'new single system' of patriarchal capitalism, a world where, as was emphasised in this and the previous chapter, the old shackles have been replaced by slippery silken ties that nonetheless bind.

It has been suggested that the concept of the 'new single system' may be a useful theoretical optic through which to explore women's health. It is proposed particularly because, dynamic though it is, much of current feminism gives little attention to health issues. In this respect I would like to repeat and support the assertion of Ellen Lewin and Virginia Olesen, quoted in the introduction to this book, that health 'permits the revelation of those elements of western cultures which bear most directly on the construction of gender and its consequences for women, men, and the larger social order' (1985: 19). Health is an important vehicle for feminists to explore the ways in which women's lives are entangled in a social economy that seemingly offers endless (liberatory) possibilities, but positions them in complex and contradictory ways that do not necessarily benefit their health. Thinking of women's health (and also men's health for that matter) through the optic of the 'new single system' reveals several things. Above all, the rigid orthodoxies of the past are breaking down, as is discernible in juxtapositions of diversity and binary difference that co-exist and necessarily feed off each other with significant, but as yet largely unexplored, implications for health. It has been argued that a new fabric of life is being woven out of contradictory impulses that themselves resist a final suturing. As the weft and weave of life is spun, it generates conflicted spaces that contain the potential for both liberatory and oppressive practices. It is women's (and men's) lives within these spaces that need to be explored in order to develop an understanding of their health.

Notes

1 Recovering gender and health in history

1 This sequestration has provided fertile ground for the claim that many prominent nineteenth-century women, such as Florence Nightingale, feigned long-term illness in order to avoid trivial domestic and social responsibilities and to create a space for intellectual work (e.g. Woodham-Smith 1950).

2 This was not 'mere translation', of course. Martineau wrote that her method was to study as she 'went along, the subjects of my author'. 'Being thus secure of what I was about, I simply set up the volume on a little desk before me, glanced over at a page or a paragraph, and set down its meaning in the briefest and simplest way I could' (Martineau 1877: 391). Her volume reduced Comte's 4,700 pages to 1,000.

3 It should come as no surprise that Alexis de Tocqueville's *Democracy in America* (1967 [1835, 1840]) is far more likely to be chosen for discussion of mid-nineteenth-century American politics and institutions than Martineau's *Society in America* (1962 [1836/1837]), despite what some regard as the methodological superiority of Martineau's account (Hill 2003). For example, in *Origins and Growth of Sociology*, J. H. Abraham (1973) praises de Tocqueville for his 'acute observation' and eulogises him as a 'supreme sociologist'. By contrast, Martineau is mentioned only as Comte's translator.

4 Of course, the phrase 'life, liberty and the pursuit of happiness' appears in the US Declaration of Independence, signed in 1776.

5 Martineau felt that the need for her informants to speak close to her ear encouraged their confidence and generated a more frank account of their lives. She also associated her inability to hear and participate in casual conversation with her use of observation as a method (although she did instruct her companion, Louisa Jeffrey, to listen and make reports to her). She was one of the earliest sociologists to study disability (Deegan 2003).

6 Comte's law of the development of human knowledge identifies three stages: the theological, the metaphysical and the positivistic (Comte 1896 [1853]).

7 Lester Ward (1841–1913) was the first president of the American Sociological Society (now the American Sociological Association). He is credited with developing a controversial evolutionary 'gynaecocentric' theory of the development of society (see discussions in Finlay 1999; Palmeri 1983).

8 Gilman's 'Our Androcentric Culture' was serialised in *The Forerunner*, a commercial journal (funded by advertisements and subscriptions) that Gilman edited between 1901 and 1916. It contained only her own writing and responses to readers' letters. The first 18 parts, published between 1901 and 1910 can be found at www.fullbooks.com/the-forerunner.html. The quotations in this chapter are taken from this website (accessed 7 August 2007).

9   Van contrasts to the character of Terry, who never learns to see things differently. He rapes his new wife when she refuses his sexual advances and is banished from herland (Gilman 1998 [1915]).

10 *The Forerunner*, www.fullbooks.com/the-forerunner.html (accessed 7 August 2007).

11 *The Forerunner*, www.fullbooks.com/the-forerunner.html (accessed 7 August 2007).

12 The American Medical Association, which previously had forbidden physicians to breach patient confidentiality, changed its position in the first decade of the twentieth century in response to the public health risk of syphilis. A 1912 revision of its ethical code now permitted physicians to break confidentiality to protect a healthy individual at risk (Cutter 2001).

13 By chastity she means abstinence from extramarital sexual relations.

14 'Classes' here should be taken to mean groups rather than social classes.

2   Making connections

1   This does not mean that all male sociologists were blind to sexism. See, for example, David Morgan's (1975) discussion of his desire to provide, as he put it, a corrective to the sexist bias in sociology by including the work of 'women's liberation authors and radical feminists' in his study of the family, and also the trepidation with which he did this. Similarly, Robert Connell (now Raewyn Connell) recounts the tensions of pursing a feminist agenda as a male head of a sociology department in the mid-to-late 1970s (Connell 1997).

2   Many of these clinics sprung up in the wake of *Roe vs Wade*, the landmark United Supreme Court case of 1973, which deemed abortion a fundamental right under the US Constitution. The central upholding was that abortions are permissible up until the point where the foetus becomes viable, which was placed at between twenty-four and twenty-eight weeks.

3   A timeline and details of various editions can be viewed at www.ourbodiesourselves.org/about/timeline.asp (accessed 26 August 2007).

4   I will refer to medical sociology in the discussion rather than the now more familiar sociology of health and illness, or sociology of health, because this was common terminology until around the 1990s. It should be noted that feminist sociologists' concern that health and health care were about more than medicine or the medical profession – that is, their recognition that much health care took place outside the formal health system – was instrumental in prompting this change in nomenclature (see Stacey 1988).

5   Despite its emphasis on the interrelations between 'public issues' of social structure and 'personal troubles', Wright Mill's 'sociological imagination' is decidedly *un*imaginative in its failure to make any reference to women.

6   For example, in their study of the professional socialisation of nurses in the US, Virginia Olesen and Elvi Waik Whittaker (1968) were concerned to promote the methodology of participant observation rather than a feminist interpretation of nurses' experience.

7   A charitable interpretation is that Bloom's focus on medical sociology's institutional development – a domain from which women have been historically excluded – rather than its intellectual history, may partially account for his inattention. Even so, women's absence from positions of influence needs to be explicitly recognised as such, rather than treated with silence.

3   Women and health status

1   It is interesting to note that although Waldron's (1976) article is entitled 'Why do women live longer than men?', the focus is heavily upon men's 'negative'

behaviour and why they die at younger ages (rather than the life-enhancing effects of women's presumably more 'positive' behaviour).

5 Thinking again about sex, gender and health

1 This discussion on gender-specific medicine draws upon currently unpublished joint work with Anne Hammarström.

6 The making of women's health

1 Between 1989 and 2006, The Portman Group ran campaigns to 'encourage responsible drinking'. This arm of its work was transferred to a new charity, The Drinkaware Trust, in late 2006. The Drinkaware Trust is supported by the Wine and Spirit Trade Association, which provides, among other things, consumer intelligence such as trends in consumer behaviour, shopping habits and so on to its members, who are, for example, merchants, distillers and wine growers.
2 Swedish snus is made from coarsely or finely ground tobacco, salt, water and aromatic substances.
3 Swedish Match is a global group with five product categories: snus/snuff, cigars, chewing tobacco, pipe tobacco, and matches. See www.swedishmatch.com.

7 Health in transition

1 Here, life expectancy refers to the average number of years that a new-born baby would survive if he or she experiences the age-specific mortality rates for that time period throughout her or his life (ONS 2007).
2 Healthy life expectancy is defined as the expected number of years lived in 'good' or 'fairly good' health and is calculated using life expectancy and self-assessed general health data (ONS 2007).
3 In Britain, the Department of Health advises that consumption of three to four units of alcohol a day for men and two to three units a day for women should not lead to significant health risks (ONS 2007).
4 Sweden has a restrictive policy on alcohol sales based on state monopoly retail stores. However, sales of alcohol have been rising in restaurants and pubs (Helmersson Bergmark 2004)
5 There is, however, some indication of a decline in the male suicide rate over recent years. Thus for England and Wales, age-standardised rates declined from 152 per million in 1998 to 125 per million in 2004. Rates for women have remained more stable at about 41 per million since 2001 (ONS 2006b).

References

Aapola, S., Gonick, M. and Harris, A. (2005) *Young Femininity. Girlhood, Power and Change*, Basingstoke: Palgrave.

Abraham, J. H. (1973) *Origins and Growth of Sociology*, Harmondsworth: Penguin.

Abrams, P., Deem, R., Finch, J. and Rock, P. (eds) (1981) *Practice and Progress: British Sociology 1850–1980*, London: George Allen & Unwin.

AIHW (Australian Institute of Health and Welfare) (2006) *Australia's Health 2006*, Canberra: AIHW.

Albrecht, G. and Higgins, P. (eds) (1979) *Health, Illness and Medicine. A Reader in Medical Sociology*, Chicago, IL: Rand NcNally.

Alexander, M. and Mohanty, C. T. (1997) 'Introduction: genealogies, legacies, movements', in M. Alexander and C. Mohanty (eds) *Feminist Genealogies, Colonial Legacies, Democratic Futures (Rethinking Gender)*, London: Routledge, pp. xiii–xlii.

Amos, A. and Haglund, M. (2000) 'From social taboo to "torch of freedom": the marketing of cigarettes to women', *Tobacco Control*, 9: 3–8.

Annandale, E. (1988) 'How midwives accomplish natural birth: managing risk and balancing expectations', *Social Problems*, 35 (2): 95–110.

Annandale, E. (1998a) *The Sociology of Health and Medicine*, Cambridge: Polity Press.

Annandale, E. (1998b) 'Health, illness and the politics of gender', in D. Field and S. Taylor (eds) *Perspectives in the Sociology of Health and Illness*, Oxford: Blackwell Scientific, pp. 115–33.

Annandale, E. (2003) 'Gender and health status', in S. Williams, L. Birke and G. Bendelow (eds) *Debating Biology*, London: Routledge, pp. 85–95.

Annandale, E. (2007) 'Assembling Harriet Martineau's gender and health jigsaw', *Women's Studies International Forum*, 30 (4): 355–66.

Annandale, E. and Clark, J. (1996) 'What is gender? Feminist theory and the sociology of human reproduction', *Sociology of Health and Illness*, 18 (1): 17–44.

Annandale, E. and Clark, J. (1997) 'A reply to Rona Campbell and Sam Porter', *Sociology of Health and Illness*, 19 (4): 521–32.

Annandale, E. and Field, D. (2007) 'Gender differences in health', in S. Taylor and D. Field (eds) *Sociology of Health and Health Care*, 4th edn, Oxford: Blackwell, pp. 93–112.

Annandale, E., Harvey, J., Cavers, D. and Dixon-Woods, M. (2007) 'Gender and access to healthcare in the UK: a critical interpretive synthesis of the literature', *Evidence and Policy*, 3 (4): 463–86.

Arber, S., McKinlay, R., Adams, A., Marceau, L., Link, C. and O'Donnell, A. (2006) 'Patient characteristics and inequalities in doctors' diagnosis and management strategies relating to CHD: a video-simulation experiment', *Social Science & Medicine*, 62 (1): 103–15.

Archer Mann, S. and Huffman, D. J. (2005) 'The decentering of second wave feminism and the rise of the third wave', *Science and Society*, 69 (1): 56–91.

Arditti, R., Duelli Klein, R. and Minden, S. (eds) (1984) *Test-Tube Women*, London: Pandora Press.

Arnot, M., David, M. and Weiner, G. (1999) *Closing the Gender Gap. Postwar Education and Social Change*, Cambridge: Polity Press.

Aschenbrand, P. (2006) *The Only Bush I Trust is my Own*, London: Corgi.

Astell, M. (2002 [1694]) *A Serious Proposal to the Ladies*. Parts I and II (ed. Patricia Springborg), Ormskirk: Broadview Press.

Badinter, E. (2006) *Dead End Feminism*, trans. J. Borossa, Cambridge: Polity Press.

Bailin, M. (1994) *The Sickroom in Victorian Fiction*, Cambridge: Cambridge University Press.

Baker, A., Griffiths, C. and Wheller, L. (2006) 'Trends in premature mortality in England and Wales, 1950–2004', *Health Statistics Quarterly*, 31: 34–41.

Balsamo, A. (1996) *Technologies of the Gendered Body. Reading Cyborg Women*, London: Duke University Press.

Banks, J. A. (1970) *Marxist Sociology in Action*, London: Faber & Faber.

Banks, O. (1981) *Faces of Feminism. A Study of Feminism as a Social Movement*, Oxford: Martin Robertson.

Banks, O. (1999) 'Some reflections on gender, sociology and women's history', *Women's History Review*, 8 (3): 401–10.

Barker, L. D. and Allen, S. (1976) 'Introduction', in L. D. Barker and S. Allen (eds) *Dependence and Exploitation in Work and Marriage*, London: Longman, pp. 1–20.

Barrett, M. (1991) *The Politics of Truth*, Cambridge: Polity Press.

Barrett, M. and Phillips, A. (1992) 'Words and things: materialism and method in contemporary feminist analysis', in M. Barrett and A. Phillips (eds) *Destabilising Theory*, Cambridge: Polity Press, pp. 201–19.

Bartley, M. (2004) *Health Inequality*, Cambridge: Polity Press.

Bates Dock, J. (ed.) (1998) *'The Yellow Wallpaper' and the History of its Publication and Reception. A Critical and Documentary Casebook*, University Park, PA: University of Pennsylvania Press.

Bauman, Z. (1998) *Work, Consumerism and the New Poor*, Buckingham: Open University Press.

Bauman, Z. (2001) *The Individualized Society*, Oxford: Polity Press.

Bauman, Z. (2002) 'Individually, together', in U. Beck and E. Beck-Gernsheim (eds) *Individualization*, London: Sage, pp. xiv–xix.

Baumgardner, J. and Richards, A. (2000) *Manifesta. Young Women, Feminism and the Future*, New York: Farrar, Straus and Giroux.

Beck, U. (2002) 'Zombie categories: interview with Ulrich Beck'. In U. Beck and E. Beck-Gernsheim (eds) *Individualization*, London: Sage, pp. 202–13.

Beck, U. and Beck-Gernsheim, E. (2002) *Individualization*, London: Sage.

Beckett, K. (2005) 'Choosing caesarean: feminism and the politics of childbirth in the United States', *Feminist Theory*, 6 (3): 251–75.

Beer, J. (1997) *Kate Chopin, Edith Wharton and Charlotte Perkins Gilman. Studies in Short Fiction*, Houndmills, Basingstoke: Macmillan Press.

Beer, J. (1998) 'Charlotte Perkins Gilman and women's health: "the long limitation"', in V. Gough and J. Rudd (eds) *A Very Different Story. Studies on the Fiction of Charlotte Perkins Gilman*, Liverpool: Liverpool University Press, pp. 54–67.

Bell, S. (1994) 'Translating science to the people. Updating *The New Our Bodies, Ourselves*', *Women's Studies International Forum*, 17 (1): 9–18.

Bell, S. E. and Reverby, S. M. (2005) 'Vaginal politics: tensions and possibilities in *The Vagina Monologues*', *Women's Studies International Forum*, 28 (5): 430–44.

Benson, R. (2000) 'Hot tipples', *Guardian*, 12 May, available at http://lifeandhealth. guardian.co.uk/fashion/story/0,,1612390,00.html.

Berger, P. and Luckmann, T. (1966) *The Social Construction of Reality*, Garden City, NY: Doubleday.

Bird, C. and Rieker, P. (2008) *Gender and Health. The Effects of Constrained Choices and Social Policies*, New York: Cambridge University Press.

Birke, L. (1999) *Feminism and the Biological Body*, Edinburgh: Edinburgh University Press.

Birke, L. (2000) 'Sitting on the fence: biology, feminism and gender-bending environments', *Women's Studies International Forum*, 23 (5): 587–99.

Birke, L. (2003) 'Feminism and the idea of "the biological"', in S. Williams, L. Birke and G. Bendelow (eds) *Debating Biology*, London: Routledge, pp. 39–52.

Black, J. and Ong, B. N. (1986) 'Women and health courses: our bodies, our business', in C. Webb (ed.) *Feminist Practice in Women's Health Care*, Chichester: John Wiley & Sons, pp. 19–33.

Blackwell, E. (1977 [1895]) *Pioneer Work in Opening the Medical Profession to Women*, New York: Schocken Books.

Blaxter, M. (2004) *Health*, Cambridge: Polity Press.

Bloom, S. (2002) *The Word as Scalpel. A History of Medical Sociology*, Oxford: Oxford University Press.

Blunt, J. (1793) *Man-midwife Dissected; or, the Obstetric Family Instructor*, London: Samuel William Fores.

Bordo, S. (1990) 'Feminism, post-modernism, and gender-scepticism', in L. Nicholson (ed.) *Feminism/postmodernism*, London: Routledge, pp. 133–56.

Bordo, S. (1993) *Unbearable Weight: Feminism, Western Culture and the Body*, London: University of California Press.

Bordo, S. (1999) *Twilight Zones*, London: University of California Press.

Boston Women's Health Book Collective (1978) *Our Bodies, Ourselves*, London: Penguin Books.

Bostock, L. (2003) *Searching for the Solution. Women, Smoking and Inequalities in Europe*, London: Health Development Agency.

Bottomore, T. (1975) *Marxist Sociology*, London: Macmillan Press.

Bottomore, T. and Goode, P. (1983) (eds) *Readings in Marxist Sociology*, Oxford: Clarendon Press.

Bowlby, J. (1951) *Child Care and the Growth of Love*, Harmondsworth: Penguin Books.

Bradley, H. (2007) *Gender*, Cambridge: Polity Press.

Braidotti, R. (2002) *Metamorphosis. Towards a Materialist Theory of Becoming*, Cambridge: Polity Press.

Brighton Women in Science Group (1980) 'Technology in the lying-in room', in L. Birke, W. Faulkner, S. Best, D. Janson-Smith and K. Overfield (eds) *Alice Through the Microscope. The Power of Science Over Women's Lives*, London: Virago, pp. 165–81.

British Sociological Association (1977) *Sociology Without Sexism. A Sourcebook*, London: BSA.

Bronholm, H. (n.d.) 'Swedish snuff – not just for men', available at www.sweden.se/templates/cs/Article____13429.aspx (accessed 13 October 2006).

Brook, B. (1999) *Feminist Perspectives on the Body*, London: Longman.

Brooke, C. (1999) *Jane Austen: Illusion and Reality*, Cambridge: D. S. Brewer.

Brown, G. and Harris, T. (1978) *Social Origins of Depression*, London: Tavistock.

Brown, W. (1995) *States of Injury. Power and Freedom in Late Modernity*, Princeton, NJ: Princeton University Press.

Budgeon, S. (2001) 'Emergent feminist(?) identities', *European Journal of Women's Studies*, 8 (1): 7–28.

Busfield, J. (1996) *Men, Women and Madness*, London: Macmillan.

Butler, J. (1990) *Gender Trouble. Feminism and the Subversion of Identity*, London: Routledge.

Butler, J. (2004) *Undoing Gender*, London: Routledge.

Caine, B. (1997) *English Feminism, 1780–1980*, Oxford: Oxford University Press.

Campbell, R. and Porter, S. (1997) 'Feminist theory and the sociology of childbirth: a response to Ellen Annandale and Judith Clark', *Sociology of Health and Illness*, 19 (3); 348–58.

Canadian Institute for Health Information (2003) *Women's Health Surveillance Report*, Ottawa: Canadian Institute for Health Information.

Cancer Research UK (2007) 'Smokeless tobacco and cancer', available at www.info.cancerresearchuk.org/healthyliving/smokingandtobacco/smokelesstobacco/ (accessed 12 August, 2007).

Carden, M. L. (1974) *The New Feminist Movement*, New York: Russell Sage Foundation.

Carrigan, T., Connell, B. and Lee, J. (1987) 'Hard and heavy: toward a new sociology of masculinity', in M. Kaufman (ed.) *Beyond Patriarchy*, New York: Oxford University Press, pp. 139–92.

Cealey Harrison, W. and Hood-Williams, J. (2002) *Beyond Sex and Gender*, London: Sage.

Chanter, T. (2000) 'Gender aporias', *Signs* 25 (4): 1237–41.

Charles, N. (2002) *Gender in Modern Britain*, Oxford: Oxford University Press.

Chase, K. (1984) *Eros and Psyche*, London: Methuen.

Chen, Y., Subramanian, S., Acevedo-Garcia, D. and Kawachi, I. (2005) 'Women's status and depressive symptoms: a multilevel analysis', *Social Science & Medicine*, 60 (1): 49–60.

Chenet, L. (2000) 'Gender and socio-economic inequalities in mortality in central and Eastern Europe', in E. Annandale and K. Hunt (eds) *Gender Inequalities in Health*, Buckingham: Open University Press, pp. 182–210.

Cixous, H. and Clément, C. (1986) *The Newly Born Woman*, trans. B. Wing, Manchester: Manchester University Press.

Clarke, A. (1995) 'Modernity, postmodernity, and reproductive processes, ca. 1890–1990, or "mommy, where do cyborgs come from anyway?"', in C. Gray with J. Figueroa-Sameroa and S. Mentor (eds) *The Cyborg Handbook*, London: Routledge.

Clarke, A. and Olesen, V. (1999) 'Revising, diffracting, acting', in A. Clarke and V. Olesen (eds) *Revisioning Women, Health, and Healing*, London: Routledge, pp. 3–48.

Clarke, A. J. (2000) ' "As seen on TV": design and domestic economy', in M. Andrews and M. M. Talbot (eds) *All the World and Her Husband. Women in Twentieth-century Consumer Culture*, London: Cassell, pp. 146–61.

Cockerham, W. (2000) 'Health lifestyles in Russia', *Social Science & Medicine*, 51 (9): 1313–24.

Cocks, J. (1988) 'Wordless emotions: some critical reflections on radical feminism', *Politics and Society*, 13 (1): 1–26.

Colapinto, J. (2000) *As Nature Made Him*, London: Quartet Books.

Coleman, D. (2000) 'Population and family', in A. H. Halsey and J. Webb (eds) *Twentieth-century British Social Trends*, Basingstoke: Macmillan, pp. 27–93.

Comaroff, J. (1977) 'Conflicting paradigms of pregnancy: managing ambiguity in ante-natal encounters', in A. Davis and G. Horobin (eds) *Medical Encounters*, London: Croom Helm, pp. 115–34.

Comte, A. (1830–42) *Cours de Philosophie Positive*. Paris: Bachelier.

Comte, A. (1896 [1853]) *The Positive Philosophy of Auguste Comte* (trans. H. Martineau), London: George Bell & Sons.

Connell, R. W. (1995) *Masculinities*, Cambridge: Polity Press.

Connell, R. W. (1997) 'Long and winding road', in B. Laslett and B. Thorne (eds) *Feminist Sociology. Life Histories of a Movement*, New Brunswick, NJ: Rutgers University Press, pp. 151–64.

Connolly, C. K. (2002) 'Letter', *British Medical Journal*, 323: 1014–15, available at www.bmj.com/cgi/eletters/323/7320/1014.

Conrad, P. (2007) *The Medicalization of Society*, Baltimore, MD: The Johns Hopkins University Press.

Conrad, P. and Kern, R. (eds) (1981) *The Sociology of Health and Illness. Critical Perspectives*, New York: St Martin's Press.

Coote, A. and Campbell, B. (1987) *Sweet Freedom*, 2nd edn, Oxford: Blackwell.

Cooter, R. (1991) 'Dichotomy and denial: mesmerism, medicine and Harriet Martineau', in M. Benjamin (ed.) *Science and Sensibility. Gender and Scientific Enquiry, 1780–1945*, Oxford: Blackwell, pp. 144–73.

Corea, G. (1985) *The Hidden Malpractice. How American Medicine Mistreats Women*, updated edition, New York: Harper Colophon Books.

Cornell, D. (1991) *Beyond Accommodation*, London: Routledge.

Cornwell, J. (1984) *Hard Earned Lives*, London: Routledge/Tavistock.

Coward, R. (2000) *Sacred Cows. Is Feminism Relevant to the New Millennium?*, London: HarperCollins.

Crompton, R. (2006a) *Employment and the Family. The Reconfiguration of Work and Family Life in Contemporary Societies*, Cambridge: Polity Press.

Crompton, R. (2006b) 'Gender and work', in K. Davis, M. Evans and J. Lorber (eds) *Handbook of Gender and Women's Studies*, London: Sage, pp. 161–78.

Cutter, M. J. (2001) 'The writer as doctor: new medical models of medical discourse in Charlotte Perkins Gilman's later fiction', *Literature and Medicine*, 20 (2): 151–82.

Dalla Costa, M. and James, S. (1995 [1972]) 'The power of women and the subversion of the community', in E. Malos (ed.) *The Politics of Housework*, London: Allen & Busby, pp. 160–87.

Daly, M. (1984) *Pure Lust: Elemental Feminist Philosophy*, London: The Women's Press.

Daly, M. (1993) *Outercourse. The Be-dazzling Voyage*, London: The Women's Press.

David, D. (1987) *Intellectual Women and Victorian Patriarchy*, Ithaca, NY: Cornell University Press.

Davidoff, L. (1995) *Worlds Between: Historical Perspectives on Gender and Class*, Cambridge: Polity Press.

Davis, A. and Horobin, G. (eds) (1977) *Medical Encounters*, London: Croom Helm.

Davis, K. (2002a) 'Feminist body/politics as world traveller. Translating *Our Bodies, Ourselves*', *European Journal of Women's Studies*, 9 (3): 223–47.

Davis, K. (2002b) '"A dubious equality": men, women and cosmetic surgery', *Body and Society*, 8 (1): 49–65.

Davis, K. (2007a) 'Reclaiming women's bodies: colonialist trope or critical epistemology?', in C. Shilling (ed.) *Embodying Sociology: Retrospect, Progress and Prospects* (Sociological Review Monograph Series), Oxford: Blackwell/The Sociological Review, pp. 50–64.

Davis, K. (2007b) *The Making of Our Bodies Ourselves: How Feminism Travelled Across Borders*, Durham, NC: Duke University Press.

Day, K., Gough, B. and McFadden. M. (2004) '"Warning! Alcohol can seriously damage your health". A discourse analysis of recent British newspaper coverage of women and drinking', *Feminist Media Studies*, 4 (2): 166–83.

de Lauretis, T. (1987) *Technologies of Gender*, London: Macmillan.

Dearey, M. (2006) 'Betty Freidan: a tribute', *Sociological Research Online*, 11 (3), available at www.swetswise.com/eAccess/viewToc.do?titleID=188303&yevoID=1764024 (accessed 12 August, 2007).

Deegan, M. J. (1997) 'Introduction: Gilman's sociological journey from *Herland* to *Ourland*', in M. J. Deegan and M. R. Hill (eds) *With Her in Ourland. Sequel to Herland*, London: Greenwood Press, pp. 1–57.

Deegan, M. J. (2003) 'Making lemonade: Harriet Martineau on being deaf', in M. Hill and S. Hoecker-Drysdale (eds), *Harriet Martineau. Theoretical and Methodological Perspectives,* London: Routledge, pp. 41–58.

Deem, R. (1996) 'Border territories: a journey through sociology, education and women's studies', *British Journal of Sociology of Education*, 17 (1): 5–19.

Delamont, S. (2001) *Changing Women, Unchanged Men?*, Buckingham: Open University Press.

Delamont, S. (2003) *Feminist Sociology*, London: Sage.

Delphy, C. (1984) *Close to Home. A Materialist Analysis of Women's Oppression*, London: Hutchinson.

Delphy, C. (1993) 'Rethinking sex and gender', *Women's Studies International Forum*, 16 (1): 1–9.

Derrida, J. (1982) *Margins of Philosophy*, trans. A. Bass, London: Harvester Press.

DHHS (Department of Health and Human Services) (2001) *Women and Smoking*, Rockville, MD: DHSS.

Di Stefano, C. (1990) 'Dilemmas of difference: feminism, modernity, and postmodernism', in L. Nicholson (ed.) *Feminism/postmodernism*, London: Routledge, pp. 63–82.

Diamond, J. and Sigmundson, K. (1997) 'Sex reassignment at birth: long-term review and clinical applications', *Archives of Paediatric and Adolescent Medicine*, 151 (May): 298–304.

Dickason, R. (2000) *British Television Advertising*, Luton: University of Luton Press.

Dickens, P. (2000) *Social Darwinism*, Buckingham: Open University Press.

Dingwall, R., Heath, C., Reid, M. and Stacey, M. (eds) (1977) *Health Care and Health Knowledge*, London: Croom Helm.

DoH (Department of Health) (2004) *Health Survey for England*, London: DoH.

DoH (Department of Health) (2007) *Health Profile of England 2007*, London: DoH.

Donnison, J. (1977) *Midwives and Medical Men: A History of the Struggle for the Control of Childbirth*, London: Heinemann Educational.

Downer, C. (1972) 'Covert sex discrimination against women as medical patients', address to the American Psychological Association Meeting, Hawaii, September 1972. Available on the CWLU Herstory website at www.cwluherstory.com/CWLU Archive/womanpatient1.html (accessed 9 September, 2003).

Doyal, L. with Pennell, I. (1979) *The Political Economy of Health*, Boston, MA: South End Press.

Doyal, L. (1995) *What Makes Women Sick. Gender and the Political Economy of Health*, London: Macmillan.

Doyal, L. (2001) 'Sex, gender and health: the need for a new approach', *British Medical Journal*, 323: 1061–3.

Doyal, L. (2003) 'Sex and gender: the challenges for epidemiologists', *International Journal of Health Services*, 33 (3): 569–79.

Doyal, L. (2006) 'Sex, gender and medicine', in D. Kelleher, J. Gabe and G. Williams (eds) *Challenging Medicine*, 2nd edn, London: Routledge, pp. 146–61.

Dreifus, C. (ed.) (1978) *Seizing Our Bodies. The Politics of Women's Health*, New York: Vintage Books.

Duffin, L. (1978) 'The conspicuous consumptive: the woman as an invalid', in S. Delamont and L. Duffin (eds) *The Nineteenth Century Woman*, London: Croom Helm, pp. 26–56.

Dumit, J. and Davis-Floyd, R. (1998) 'Cyborg babies. Children of the third millennium', in R. Davis-Floyd and J. Dumit (eds) *Cyborg Babies. From Techno-sex to Techno-tots*, London: Routledge, 1–18.

Durkheim, E. (1968 [1893]) *The Division of Labour in Society*, New York: Free Press.

Durkheim, E. (1970 [1897]) *Suicide*, London: Routledge.

Ebert, T. (1988) 'The romance of patriarchy: ideology, subjectivity, and postmodern feminist cultural theory', *Cultural Critique*, 10 (Fall): 19–57.

Ebert, T. (1991) 'Writing in the political: resistance (post)modernism', *Legal Studies Forum*, 9 (4): 291–303.

Ebert, T. (1993) 'Ludic feminism, the body, performance, and labor: bringing *materialism* back into feminist studies', *Cultural Critique*, 23 (Winter): 5–50.

Ebert, T. (1996) *Ludic Feminism and After. Postmodernism, Desire and Labor in Late Capitalism*, Ann Arbor, MI: University of Michigan Press.

Eckman, A. (1998) 'Beyond "the Yentl Syndrome": making women visible in post-1990 women's health discourse', in P. Treichler, L. Cartwright and C. Penley (eds) *The Visible Woman*, London: New York University Press, pp. 130–68.

EHEMU (European Health Expectancy Monitoring Unit) (2005) *Are We Living Longer, Healthier Lives in the EU?*, Montpelier: EHEMU Technical Report 2.

Ehrenreich, B. and English, D. (1978) *For Her Own Good. 150 Years of Experts' Advice to Women*, New York: Anchor Books.

Eisenstein, Z. (1981) *The Radical Future of Liberal Feminism*, Boston, MA: Northeastern University Press.

Eisenstein. Z. (1988) *The Female Body and the Law*, London: University of California Press.

Elam, D. (1994) *Feminism and Deconstruction*, London: Routledge.

Eldridge, J. (1980) *Recent British Sociology*, London: Macmillan.

Eliot, G. (1855) 'Margaret Fuller and Mary Wollstonecraft', reprinted in R. Ashton (ed.) (2000) *George Elliot. Selected Writings*, Oxford: Oxford University Press, pp. 180–6.

Elliott, S. (2007) 'A new Camel brand is dressed to the nines', *New York Times*, 15 February, available at www.nytimes.com/2007/02/15/business/media/15adco. html (accessed 2 April, 2007).

Emerson, J. (1970) 'Behavior in private places: sustaining definitions of reality in gynaecological examinations', in H. Dreitzel (ed.) *Recent Sociology*, London: Collier-Macmillan, pp. 73–97.

Emslie, C. (2005) 'Women, men and coronary heart disease: review of the qualitative literature', *Journal of Advanced Nursing*, 51 (4): 382–95.

Emslie, C., Hunt, K. and Macintyre, S. (1999) 'Gender differences in minor morbidity among full time employees of a British University', *Journal of Epidemiology and Community Health*, 53 (8): 465–75.

Engels, F. (1972 [1844]) *Origin of the Family, Private Property and the State*. London: Lawrence & Wishart.

Ensler, E. (2001) *The Vagina Monologues*, London: Virago.

EOC (Equal Opportunities Commission) (2006) *Facts About Women and Men in Great Britain*, London: EOC.

Epstein, J. (1990) 'Either/or – neither/both: sexual ambiguity and the ideology of gender', *Genders*, 7 (Spring): 99–142.

Ettorre, E. (1997) *Women and Alcohol. A Private Pleasure or a Public Problem?*, London: The Women's Press.

Ettorre, E. (2002) *Reproductive Genetics, Gender and the Body*, London: Routledge.

European Commission (2000) *Report on the State of Young People's Health in the European Union*. Brussels: EU.

Evans, M. (2003) *Gender and Social Theory*, Buckingham: Open University Press.

Faludi, S. (1991) *Backlash. The Undeclared War Against American Women*, New York: Anchor Books.

Faludi, S. (1999) *Stiffed. The Betrayal of Modern Man*, London: Vintage.

Farquhar, D. (1996) *The Other Machine. Discourse and Reproductive Technologies*, London: Routledge.

Fausto-Sterling, A. (2003) 'The problem with sex/gender and nature/nurture', in S. Williams, L. Birke and G. Bendelow (eds) *Debating Biology*, London: Routledge, pp. 123–32.

Fausto-Sterling, A. (2005) 'The bare bones of sex: part 1 – sex and gender', *Signs* 30 (5): 1491–526.

Featherstone, M. (2007) *Consumer Culture and Postmodernism*, 2nd edn, London: Sage.

Ferguson, M. (1983) *Forever Feminine. Women's Magazines and the Cult of Femininity*, London: Heinemann.

Field, D. and Blakemore, K. (2007) 'Ethnicity and health', in S. Taylor and D. Fields (eds) *Sociology of Health and Health Care*, 4th edn, Oxford: Blackwell, pp. 69–92.

Finlay, B. (1999) 'Lester Ward as a sociologist of gender: a new look at his sociological work', *Gender and Society*, 13 (2): 251–65.

Finney, A. (2006) 'Domestic violence, sexual assault and stalking: findings from the 2004/05 British Crime Survey', Online Report 12/06, London: Home Office, available at www.homeoffice.gov.uk/rds/pdfs04/hors276.pdf.

Firestone, S. (1971) *The Dialectic of Sex. The Case for Feminist Revolution*, London: Jonathan Cape.

Firestone, S. (1998) *Airless Spaces*, New York: Semiotext(e).

Fisher, S. (1984) 'Doctor-patient communication: a social and micro-political performance', *Sociology of Health & Illness*, 6 (1): 1–29.

Fisher, S. and S. Groce (1985) 'Doctor-patient negotiation of cultural assumptions', *Sociology of Health & Illness*, 7 (3): 342–74.

Flax, J. (1990) *Thinking Fragments. Psychoanalysis, Feminism and Postmodernism in the Contemporary West*, Oxford: University of California Press.

Foley, L. and Faircloth, C. (2003) 'Medicine as discursive resource: legitimation in the work narratives of midwives', *Sociology of Health & Illness*, 25 (2): 165–84.

Frankfort, E. (1972) *Vaginal Politics*. New York: Quadrangle Books.

Frawley, M. (1997) '"A prisoner to the couch": Harriet Martineau, invalidism, and self-representation', in D. T. Mitchell and S. L. Snyder (eds) *The Body and Physical Difference. Discourses of Disability*, Ann Arbor, MI: The University of Michigan Press, pp. 174–88.

Frawley, M. (2004) *Invalidism and Identity in Nineteenth-Century Britain*, London: University of Chicago Press.

Freeman, J. (1973) 'The origins of the women's liberation movement', *American Journal of Sociology*, 78 (4): 792–811.

Freidman, E. (1978) *Labour: Clinical Evaluation and Management,* 2nd edn, New York: Appleton-Century-Crofts.

Freidson, E. (1970) *Profession of Medicine*, Chicago, IL: Chicago University Press.

Friedan, B. (1963) *The Feminine Mystique*, New York: Dell.

Friedan, B. (1976) *It Changed My Life*, New York: Dell.

Friedan, B. (1981) *The Second Stage*, New York: Summit Books.

Friedan, B. (1993) *Fountain of Age*, New York: Simon & Schuster.

Frost, L. (2001) *Young Women and the Body*, London: Palgrave.

Fuat Firat, A. (1994) 'Gender and consumption: transcending the feminine?', in J. Arnold Costa (ed.) *Gender Issues and Consumer Behavior*, London: Sage, pp. 205–27.

Fuller, S. (2006) *The New Sociological Imagination*, London: Sage.

Fuss, D. (1989) *Essentially Speaking. Feminism, Nature and Difference*, London: Routledge.

Fuss, D. (1991) *Inside/out*, London: Routledge.

Gardiner, J. (1976) 'Domestic labour in capitalist society', in D. Leonard Barker and S. Allen (eds) *Dependence and Exploitation in Work and Marriage*, London: Longman, pp. 109–20.

Gartner, C., Hall, W. D., Vos, T., Bertram, M. Y., Wallace, A. L. and Lim, S. S. (2007) 'Assessment of Swedish snus for tobacco harm reduction: an epidemiological modelling study', *The Lancet*, 369: 2010–14.

Gaskell, E. (1985 [1853]) *Ruth*, Oxford: Oxford University Press.

Gatens, M. (1983) 'A critique of the sex/gender distinction', in J. Allen and P. Patton (eds) *Beyond Marxism*, Leichardt: Intervention Publishing, pp. 143–60.

Gavron, H. (1966) *The Captive Wife: Conflicts of Housebound Mothers*, Harmonds-worth: Pelican Books.

Gélis, J. (1991) *History of Childbirth*, Cambridge: Polity Press.

Genz, S. (2006) 'Third Way/ve', *Feminist Theory*, 7 (3): 333–53.

Gerhardt, U. (1989) *Ideas about Illness. An Intellectual and Political History of Medical Sociology*, London: Macmillan.

GHS (General Household Survey) (2004) *General Household Survey 2004*, available at www.statistics.gov.uk/ghs.

Gibson-Graham, J. K. (1996) *The End of Capitalism (As We Know It). A Feminist Critique of Political Economy*, Oxford: University of California Press.

Giddens, A. (1991) *Modernity and Self Identity*, Cambridge: Polity Press.

Giddens, A. (1992) *The Transformation of Intimacy*, Cambridge: Polity Press.

Gilleard, C. and Higgs, P. (2000) *Cultures of Ageing*, Harlow: Pearson Education.

Gilman, C. P. (1908) 'A suggestion on the negro problem', *American Journal of Sociology*, 14 (1): 78–85.

Gilman, C. P. (1913a) 'Why I wrote the Yellow Wallpaper', reprinted in J. Bates Dock (ed.) (1998) *'The Yellow Wallpaper' and the History of its Publication and Reception. A Critical and Documentary Casebook*, University Park, PA: University of Pennsylvania Press, p. 86.

Gilman, C. P. (1913b) 'Excerpt from *The Living of Charlotte Perkins Gilman: An Autobiography*', reprinted in T. L. Erskine and C. L. Richards (eds) (1993) *The Yellow Wallpaper*, New Brunswick, NJ: Rutgers University Press, pp. 87–9.

Gilman, C. P. (1915) *Herland* (unabridged), Mineola, NY: Dover Publications.

Gilman, C. P. (1916a) 'The "nervous breakdown" of women', reprinted in T. L. Erskine and C. L. Richards (eds) (1993) *The Yellow Wallpaper*, New Brunswick, NJ: Rutgers University Press, pp. 67–75.

Gilman, C. Perkins (1916b) *With Her in Ourland. Sequel to Herland*, reprinted in M. J. Deegan and M. R. Hill (eds) (1997) *With Her in Ourland. Sequel to Herland*, London: Greenwood Press.

Gilman, C. P. (1916c) 'The vintage', reprinted in D. D. Knight (ed.) (1999) *Charlotte Perkins Gilman. Herland, The Yellow Wall-Paper and Selected Writings*, London: Penguin Books, pp. 297–304.

Gilman, C. P. (1923) 'The new generation of women', *The Current History Magazine*, pp. 731–7.

Gilman, C. P. (1963 [1935]) *The Living of Charlotte Perkins Gilman*, Madison, WI: University of Wisconsin Press.

Gilman, C. P. (1966 [1898]) *Women and Economics*, ed. Carl N. Degler, London: Harper Torchbooks.

Gilman, C. P. (1973 [1892]) *The Yellow Wallpaper*, New York: The Feminist Press.

Gjonça, A., Tomassini, C., Toson, B. and Smallwood, S. (2005) 'Sex differences in mortality, a comparison of the United Kingdom and other developed countries', *Health Statistics Quarterly*, 26: 6–16.

Goffman, E. (1979) *Gender Advertisements*, London: Macmillan.

Goode, W. (1964) *The Family*, Englewood Cliffs, NJ: Prentice Hall.

Gorman, B. K. and Ghazal Read, J. (2006) 'Gender disparities in adult health: an examination of three measures of morbidity', *Journal of Health and Social Behaviour*, 47 (June): 95–100.

Gove, W. (1972) 'Sex, marital status, and mortality', *American Journal of Sociology*, 79 (1): 45–65.

Gove, W. and Hughes, M. (1979) 'Possible causes of the apparent sex differences in physical health: an empirical investigation', *American Sociological Review*, 44: 126–46.

Grace, V. (2007) 'Beyond dualism in the life sciences: implications for a feminist critique of gender-specific medicine', *Journal of Interdisciplinary Feminist Thought*, 2 (1): 1–18.

Graham, H. (2000) 'Socio-economic change and inequalities in men and women's health in the UK', in E. Annandale and K. Hunt (eds) *Gender Inequalities in Health*, Buckingham: Open University Press, pp. 90–122.

Graham, H. and Oakley, A. (1981) 'Competing ideologies of reproduction: medical and maternal perspectives on pregnancy', in H. Roberts (ed.) *Women, Health and Reproduction*, London: Routledge/Kegan Paul, pp. 50–74.

Greer, G. (1971) *The Female Eunuch*, London: Paladin.

Grenier, A. and Hanley, J. (2007) 'Older women and frailty', *Current Sociology*, 55 (2): 211–28.

Griffin, S. (1978) *Woman and Nature: The Roaring Inside Her*, London: Harper & Row.

Griffiths, C. and Brock, A. (2003) 'Twentieth century mortality trends in England and Wales', *Health Statistics Quarterly*, 18: 5–17.

Grosz, E. (1990) 'Contemporary theories of power and subjectivity', in S. Gunew (ed.) *Feminist Knowledge: Critique and Construct*, London: Routledge, pp. 59–120.

Grosz, E. (1994) *Volatile Bodies*, Bloomington, IN: Indiana University Press.

Grosz, E. (1995) *Space, Time, and Perversion*, London: Routledge.

Guardian Unlimited (2001) 'Stressed "goddesses" cling to ladette past', *Guardian Unlimited Archive*, available at www.guardian.co.uk/Archive/Article/0,4273, 4170907,00.html (accessed 4 May, 2001).

Gupta, J. A. (2006) 'Towards transnational feminisms. Some reflections and concerns in relation to the globalisation of reproductive technologies', *European Journal of Women's Studies*, 13 (1): 23–38.

Hamilton, P. (1992) 'The Enlightenment and the birth of social science', in S. Hall and B. Gieben (eds) *Formations of Modernity*, Cambridge: Open University Press/Polity Press, pp. 17–58.

Hanson, B. (2000) 'The social construction of sex categories as problematic to biomedical research: cancer as a case in point', in J. Jacobs Kronenfeld (ed.) *Health, Illness, and Use of Care: The Impact of Social Factors*, London: JAI, pp. 53–68.

Haraway, D. (1985) 'A manifesto for cyborgs: science, technology, and socialist feminism in the 1980s', *Socialist Review*, 80: 65–108.

Haraway, D. (1997) *Modest_Witness@Second_Millennium. FemaleMan©_Meets_ Oncomouse^{TM}: Feminism and Technoscience*, London: Routledge.

Härenstam, A., Aronsson, G. and Hammarström, A. (2001) 'The future of gender inequalities in health', in P. Östlin, M. Danielsson, F. Diderichsen, A. Härenstam and G. Lindberg (eds) *Gender Inequalities in Health. A Swedish Perspective*, trans. D. Duncan, Boston, MA: Harvard University Press, pp. 269–304.

Harman, J., Graham, H., Frances, G., Inskip, H. and the SWS Study Group (2006) 'Socioeconomic gradients in smoking among young women: a British survey', *Social Science & Medicine*, 63 (11): 2791–800.

Hart, N. (1996) 'Procreation: the substance of female oppression in modern society. Part two: feminism and the spirit of capitalism', in N. Keddie (ed.) *Debating Gender, Debating Sexuality*, London: New York University Press, pp. 25–48.

Hartmann, H. (1981) 'The unhappy marriage of Marxism and feminism: toward a more progressive union', in L. Sargent (ed.) *Women and Revolution: A Discussion of the Unhappy Marriage of Marxism and Feminism*, Montreal: Black Rose Books, pp. 363–73.

Harvey, W. J. (1985) 'Introduction', in G. Eliot, *Middlemarch*, London: Penguin Books, pp. 7–22.

Helmersson Bergmark, K. (2004) 'Gender roles, family, and drinking: women at the crossroads of drinking cultures', *Journal of Family History*, 29 (3): 293–307.

Hennessy, R. (1993) *Materialist Feminism and the Politics of Discourse*, London: Routledge.

Hennessy, R. (2000) *Profit and Pleasure*, London: Routledge.

Henry, A. (2004) *Not My Mother's Sister. Generational Conflict and Third-Wave Feminism*, Bloomington, IN: Indiana University Press.

Herzlich, C. (1973) *Health and Illness: A Social Psychological Approach*, London: Academic Press.

Heywood, L. and Drake, J. (1997) 'Introduction', in L. Heywood and J. Drake (eds) *Third Wave Agenda. Being Feminist, Doing Feminism*, London: University of Minnesota Press, pp. 1–20.

Hill, B. (ed.) (1986) *The First English Feminist. Reflections Upon Marriage and Other Writings by Mary Astell*, Aldershot: Gower/Maurice Temple Smith.

Hill, M. (1980) *Charlotte Perkins Gilman. The Making of a Radical Feminist 1860–1896*, Philadelphia, PA: Temple University Press.

Hill, M. (2003) 'A methodological comparison of Harriet Martineau's *Society in America* (1837) and Alexis de Tocqueville's *Democracy in America* (1835–1840)', in M. R. Hill and S. Hoecker-Drysdale (eds) *Harriet Martineau. Theoretical and Methodological Perspectives*, London: Routledge, pp. 59–74.

Hill, M. R. and Hoecker-Drysdale, S. (2003) 'Taking Harriet Martineau seriously in the classroom and beyond', in M. R. Hill and S. Hoecker-Drysdale (eds) *Harriet Martineau. Theoretical and Methodological Perspectives*, London: Routledge, pp. 3–22.

Hilton, M. (2000) *Smoking in British Popular Culture*, Manchester: Manchester University Press.

Hoecker-Drysdale, S. (2003) 'Harriet Martineau and the positivism of Auguste Comte', in M. R. Hill and S. Hoecker-Drysdale (eds) *Harriet Martineau. Theoretical and Methodological Perspectives*, London: Routledge, pp. 169–89.

Hood-Williams, J. (1996) 'Goodbye to sex and gender', *Sociological Review*, 44 (1): 1–17.

Hopkins, S. (2002) *Girl Heroes. The New Force in Popular Culture*, Locked Bag, New South Wales: Pluto Press.

Hornblum, A. (1998) *Acres of Skin. Human Experiments at Holmesburg Prison*, London: Routledge.

Howson, A. (2005) *Embodying Gender*, London: Sage.

Hughes, C. (2002) *Women's Contemporary Lives*, London: Routledge.

Hunt, S. (2004) 'Foreword', in M. Stewart (ed.) *Pregnancy, Birth and Maternity Care. Feminist Perspectives*, London: Books for Midwives, pp. ix–x.

Inhorn, M. L. and Whittle, K. L. (2001) 'Feminism meets the "new" epidemiologies: toward an appraisal of antifeminist biases in epidemiological research on women's health', *Social Science & Medicine*, 53 (5): 553–67.

Jackson, S. (1992) 'The amazing deconstructing woman,' *Trouble and Strife*, 25 (Winter): 25–31.

Jackson, S. (1999) *Heterosexuality in Question*, London: Sage.

Jackson, S. (2001) 'Why a materialist feminism is (still) possible – and necessary', *Women's Studies International Forum*, 24 (3/4): 283–93.

Jaggar, A. (1983) *Feminist Politics and Human Nature*, Totowa, NJ: Rowman & Littlefield.

James, A. and Hockey, J. (2007) *Embodying Health Identities*, Basingstoke: Palgrave.

Jamieson, L. (1999) 'Intimacy transformed? A critical look at the "pure relationship"', *Sociology*, 33 (3): 477–94.

Johansson, S. R. (1996) 'Excess female mortality. Constructing survival during the development in Meiji Japan and Victorian England', in A. Digby and J. Stewart (eds) *Gender, Health and Welfare*, London: Routledge, pp. 32–66.

Jones, H. (2001) 'Health and reproduction', in I. Zweniger-Bargielowska (ed.) *Women in Twentieth-century Britain*, London: Longman, pp. 86–101.

Jones, J. (1981) *Bad Blood. The Tuskegee Syphilis Experiment*, London: The Free Press.

Jones, S. (2002) *The Descent of Men*, London: Little, Brown.

Jordanova, L. (1999) *Nature Displayed. Gender, Science and Medicine 1760–1820*, London: Longman.

Jump, H. D. (ed.) (1998) *Nineteenth-century Short Stories by Women. A Routledge Anthology*, London: Routledge.

Kampf, A. (2006) 'Report on the conference on "Men, Women and Medicine: A New View of the Biology of Sex/Gender Differences and Ageing" held in Berlin, 24–26th February 2006', *Philosophy, Ethics and Humanities in Medicine*, 1 (11), available at www.peh-med.com/content/1/1/11.

Kandrack, M., Grant, K. and Segall, A. (1991) 'Gender differences in health related behaviour: some unanswered questions', *Social Science & Medicine*, 32 (5): 579–90.

Kane, P. (1994) *Women's Health. From Womb to Tomb*, London: Macmillan.

Kaufert, P. (1999) 'The vanishing woman: gender and population health', in T. Pollard and S. Brin Hyatt (eds) *Sex, Gender and Health*, Cambridge: Cambridge University Press, pp. 118–36.

Kaufman, N. and Nichter, M. (2001) 'The marketing of tobacco to women: global perspectives', in J. Samet and S. Yoon (eds) *Women and the Tobacco Epidemic*, Geneva: World Health Organisation, pp. 69–98.

Kaufmann, T. (2004) 'Introducing feminism', in M. Stewart (ed.) *Pregnancy, Birth and Maternity Care. Feminist Perspectives*, London: Books for Midwives, pp. 1–10.

Kawachi, I., Kennedy, B. P., Gupta, V. and Prothrow-Stith, D. (1999) 'Women's status and the health of women and men: a view from the states', *Social Science & Medicine*, 48 (1): 21–32.

Keller, E. (1997) 'Producing petty gods: Margaret Cavendish's critique of experimental science', *English Literary History*, 64: 447–71.

Kent, J. (2000) *Social Perspectives on Pregnancy and Childbirth for Midwives, Nurses and the Caring Professions*, Buckingham: Open University Press.

Kessler, S. (1990) 'The medical construction of gender: case management of inter-sexed infants', *Signs*, 16 (1): 3–26.

Kessler, S. (1998) *Lessons from the Intersexed*, London: Rutgers University Press.

Khoury, A. and Weisman, C. (2002) 'Thinking about women's health: the case for gender sensitivity', *Women's Health Issues*, 12 (2): 61–64.

Kirby, V. (1997) *Telling Flesh. The Substance of the Corporeal*, London: Routledge.

Kirkham, M. (1983) *Jane Austen, Feminism and Fiction*, Brighton, Sussex: Harvester Press.

Kirkham, M. (1986) 'A feminist perspective in midwifery', in C. Webb (ed.) *Feminist Practice in Women's Health Care*, Chichester: Wiley, pp. 35–49.

Kitzinger, S. (1962) *The Experience of Childbirth*, London: Victor Gollancz.

Kitzinger, S. (2004) *The New Experience of Childbirth*, London: Orion.

Klein, R. (1996) '(Dead) bodies floating in cyberspace: post-modernism and the dismemberment of women', in D. Bell and R. Klein (eds) *Radically Speaking. Feminism Reclaimed*, London: Zed Books, pp. 346–58.

Klima, C. S. (2001) 'Women's health care: a new paradigm for the 21st century', *Journal of Midwifery and Women's Health*, 46 (5): 285–91.

Klumb, P. L. and Lampert, T. (2004) 'Women, work and well-being 1950–2000: a review and methodological critique', *Social Science & Medicine*, 58 (6): 1007–24.

Ko, Y., Cheng, L., Lee, C., Huang, J., Huang, M., Kao, E., Wang, H., and Lin, H. (2000) 'Chinese food cooking and lung cancer in women nonsmokers', *American Journal of Epidemiology*, 151 (2): 140–7.

Krieger, Nancy (2001) 'Theories for social epidemiology in the 21st-century: an ecosocial perspective', *International Journal of Epidemiology*, 30 (4): 668–77.

Krieger, N. (2003) 'Genders, sexes, and health: what are the connections – and why does it matter?', *International Journal of Epidemiology*, 32 (4): 652–7.

Krieger, N. and Zierler, S. (1995) 'Accounting for the health of women', *Current Issues in Public Health*, 1: 251–256.

Krieger, N. and Davey Smith, G. (2004) '"Bodies count", and body counts: social epidemiology and embodying inequality', *Epidemiological Reviews*, 26: 92–103.

Kuhlmann, E. (forthcoming) 'From women's health to gender mainstreaming and back again: linking feminist agendas and new governance in health care', in E. Annandale and E. Riska (eds) *New Connections: Towards a Gender Inclusive Approach to Women's and Men's Health* (Current Sociology Monograph), London: Sage.

Kuhlmann, E. and Babitsch, B. (2002) 'Bodies, health and gender – bridging feminist theories and women's health', *Women's Studies International Forum*, 25 (4): 433–42.

Lagro-Janssen, T. (2007) 'Sex, gender and health', *European Journal of Women's Studies*, 14 (1): 9–20.

Lahelma, E., Arber, S., Martikainen, P., Rahkonen, O. and Silventoinen, K. (2001) 'The myth of gender differences in health: social structural determinants across adult ages in Britain and Finland', *Current Sociology*, 49 (3): 31–54.

Landry, D. and MacLean, G. (1993) *Materialist Feminisms*, Oxford: Blackwell.

Lane, A. (1997) *To Herland and Beyond: The Life and Work of Charlotte Perkins Gilman*, London: University of Virginia Press.

Laqueur, T. (1990) *Making Sex*, London: Harvard University Press.

Lash, S. (2002) 'Individualization in a non-linear mode', in U. Beck and E. Beck-Gernsheim (eds) *Individualization*, London: Sage, pp. vii–xiii.

Laslett, B. and Thorne, B. (1997) 'Life histories of a movement: an introduction', in B. Laslett and B. Thorne (eds) *Feminist Sociology. Life Histories of a Movement*, New Brunswick, NJ: Rutgers University Press, pp. 1–27.

Layne, L. (2003) 'Unhappy endings: a feminist reappraisal of the women's health movement from the vantage of pregnancy loss', *Social Science & Medicine*, 56 (9): 1881–91.

Leap, N. (2004) 'Journey to midwifery through feminism: a personal account', in M. Stewart (ed.) *Pregnancy, Birth and Maternity Care. Feminist Perspectives*, London: Books for Midwives, pp. 185–200.

Legato, M. (2003a) *Eve's Rib. The New Science of Gender-Specific Medicine and How it Can Save Your Life*, New York: Random House.

Legato, M. (2003b) 'Beyond women's health. The new discipline of gender-specific medicine', *Medical Clinics of North America*, 87: 917–37.

Lehmann, J. (1994) *Durkheim and Women*, London: University of Nebraska Press.

Levy, A. (2005) *Female Chauvinist Pigs. Women and the Rise of Raunch Culture*, New York: Free Press.

Lewin, E. and Olesen, V. (1985) (eds) *Women, Health, and Healing*, London: Tavistock.

Liaw, Y., Huang, Y. and Lien, G. (2005) 'Patterns of lung cancer mortality in 23 countries: application of the age-period-cohort model', *BMC Public Health* 5: 22, available at www.biomedcentral.com/1471-2458/5/22.

Lindsay, C. (2003) 'A century of labour market change', *Labour Market Trends*, 111 (March): 133–44.

Linstead, S. (1993) 'Deconstruction in the study of organisations', in J. Hassard and M. Parker (eds) *Postmodernism and Organisations*, London: Sage, pp. 49–70.

Lloyd, G. (1993 [1984]) *The Man of Reason. 'Male' and 'Female' in Western Philosophy,* London: Routledge.

Logan, D. (2002) *The Hour and the Woman. Harriet Martineau's "Somewhat Remarkable" Life*, Dekalb, IL: Northern Illinois University Press.

Lohan, M. (2007) 'How might we understand men's health better? Integrating explanations from critical studies on men and inequalities in health', *Social Science & Medicine*, 65 (3): 493–504.

Looser, D. (1995) 'Introduction: Jane Austen and discourses of feminism', in D. Loosner (ed.) *Jane Austen and Discourses of Feminism*, Basingstoke: Macmillan, pp. 1–16.

Lorber, J. (2005) *Breaking the Bowls. Degendering and Feminist Change*, New York: W. W. Norton & Co.

Lowe, D. M. (1995) *The Body in Late-Capitalist USA*, London: Duke University Press.

Lu, T. (2007) 'Trends in gender differences in mortality in Taiwan: similarities and differences in pattern of changes by causes of death', paper presented at *Workshop on Gender and Medicine*, Tainan, Taiwan, 14 April.

Luker, K. (1975) *Taking Chances. Abortion and the Decision not to Contracept*, London: University of California Press.

Lupton, D. (2003) *Medicine as Culture*, 2nd edn, London: Sage.

Lury, C. (2002) 'From diversity to heterogeneity: a feminist analysis of the making of kinds', *Economy and Society*, 31 (4): 588–605.

McCool, W. and McCool., S. (1989) 'Feminism and nurse-midwifery', *Journal of Nurse-Midwifery*, 34 (6): 323–34.

McDonald, L. (2003) 'The Florence Nightingale-Harriet Martineau connection', in M. R. Hill and S. Hoecker-Drysdale (eds) *Harriet Martineau. Theoretical and Methodological Perspectives*, London: Routledge, pp. 153–68.

McDonough, P. and Walters, V. (2001) 'Gender and health: reassessing patterns and explanations', *Social Science & Medicine*, 52 (4): 547–59.

McDowell, L. (2003) *Redundant Masculinities*, Oxford: Blackwell.

Macintyre, S. (1977) *Single and Pregnant*, London: Croom Helm.

Macintyre, S. (1978) '"Who wants babies?" The social construction of "instincts"', in D. Leonard Barker and S. Allen (eds) *Sexual Divisions and Society: Process and Change*, London: Tavistock, pp. 150–173.

Macintyre, S., Hunt, K. and Sweeting, H. (1996) 'Gender differences in health: are things as simple as they seem?', *Social Science & Medicine*, 42 (4): 617–24.

Macintyre, S., Hunt, K. and Ford, G. (1999) 'Do women "over-report" morbidity? Men's and women's responses to structured prompting on a standard questionnaire on long standing illness', *Social Science & Medicine*, 48 (1): 89–98.

McMunn, A., Bartley, M., Hardy, R. and Kuh, D. (2006) 'Life course social roles and health in mid-life: causation or selection?', *Journal of Epidemiology and Community Health*, 60: 484–9.

McRobbie, A. (2000) *Feminism and Youth Culture*, 2nd edn, London: Macmillan.

Madoo Lengermann, P. and Niebrugge-Brantley, J. (1998) *The Women Founders*, London: McGraw-Hill.

Madoo Lengermann, P. and Niebrugge-Brantley, J. (2003) 'The meaning of "things": theory and method in Harriet Martineau's *How to Observe Morals and Manners* (1853) and Emile Durkheim's *The Rules of Sociological Method* (1895)', in M. R. Hill and S. Hoecker-Drysdale (eds) *Harriet Martineau: Theoretical and Methodological Perspectives*, London: Routledge, pp. 75–97.

Malos, E. (ed.) (1995) *The Politics of Housework*, London: Allen & Busby.

Mansfield, B. (2008) 'The social nature of natural childbirth', *Social Science & Medicine*, 66 (5): 1084–94.

Marmot, M. (2005) *Status Syndrome. How Your Social Standing Directly Affects Your Health*, London: Bloomsbury Publishing.

Marsh, B. (2004) 'The ladette takeover', *Daily Mail*, 19 January, available at www.dailymail.co.uk/pages/live/articles/health/womenfamily.html?in_article_id=206192&in_page_id=1799.

Marshall, B. (1994) *Engendering Modernity*, Cambridge: Polity Press.

Martin, E. (1987) *The Woman in the Body*, Milton Keynes: Open University Press.

Martineau, H. (1838) *How to Observe Morals and Manners*, London: Charles Knight and Co.

Martineau, H. (1844) *Letters on Mesmerism*, London: Edward Moxon.

Martineau, H. (1853) *The Positive Philosophy of Auguste Comte*, trans. H. Martineau, London: Bell.

Martineau, H. (1861) *Health, Husbandry, and Handicraft*, London: Bradbury and Evans.

Martineau, H. (1877) *Harriet Martineau's Autobiography, Vol II*, with memorials by Maria Weston Chapman, London: Smith, Elder & Co.

Martineau, H. (1962 [1836/1837]) *Society in America,* ed. S. M. Lipset, New York: Anchor Books.

Martineau, H. (2003 [1844]) *Life in the Sick-Room*, ed. M. Frawley, Ormskirk: Broadview Press.

Martineau, H. (2004 [1839]) *Deerbrook*, London: Penguin Books.

Mathieu, C. (1996) 'Sexual, sexed and sex-class identities: three ways of concep-tualising the relationship between sex and gender', in D. Leonard and L. Adkins (eds) *Sex in Question*, London: Taylor & Francis, pp. 42–71.

Matthaei, J. A. (1982) *An Economic History of Women in America*, New York: Schocken Books.

Mattel (2007) website available at www.mattel.com/our_toys/ot_barb.asp (accessed June 2007).

Mead, M. (1971 [1950]) *Male and Female*, Harmondsworth: Pelican Books.

Mechanic, D. (1978) *Medical Sociology*, 2nd edn, New York: Free Press.

Mechanic, D. (ed.) (1980) *Readings in Medical Sociology*, New York: Free Press.

Meryn, S. (2004) 'Gender quo vadis? 21 the first female century?', *Journal of Men's Health and Gender*, 1 (1): 3–7.

Michie, H. and Cahn, N. (1996) 'Unnatural births: caesarean sections in the discourse of "natural childbirth"', in C. Sargent and C. Bretnall (eds) *Gender and Health. An International Perspective*, Upper Saddle River, NJ: Prentice-Hall, pp. 44–56.

Millett, K. (1970) *Sexual Politics*, New York: Doubleday.

Mitchell, J. (1996) 'Juliet Mitchell responds to Nicky Hart,' in N. Keddie (ed.) *Debating Gender, Debating Sexuality*, London: New York University Press, pp. 49–51.

Moi, T. (1999) *What is a Woman?*, Oxford: Oxford University Press.

Monahan Lang, M. and Risman, B. J.(2006) 'Blending into equality. Family diversity and gender convergence', in K. Davis, M. Evans and J. Lorber (eds) *Handbook of Gender and Women's Studies*, London: Sage, pp. 287–303.

Money, J. and Ehrhardt, A. (1972) *Man and Woman, Boy and Girl: The Differen-tiation and Dimorphism of Gender Identity from Conception to Maturity*, Baltimore, MD: The Johns Hopkins University Press.

Morgan, D. (1975) *Social Theory and the Family*, London: Routledge/Kegan Paul.

Morgan, R. (1996) 'Light bulbs, radishes, and the politics of the 21st century', in D. Bell and R. Klein (eds) *Radically Speaking. Feminism Reclaimed*, London: Zed Books, pp. 5–8.

Morgen, S. (2002) *Into Our Own Hands. The Women's Health Movement in the United States, 1969–1990*, London: Rutgers University Press.

Moss, N. (2002) 'Gender equity and socioeconomic inequality: a framework for the patterning of women's health', *Social Science & Medicine*, 54 (5): 649–61.

Nathanson, C. (1975) 'Illness and the feminine role: a theoretical review', *Social Science & Medicine*, 9 (2): 57–62.

Nathanson, C. (1977) 'Sex, illness and medical care: a review of data, theory and method', *Social Science & Medicine*, 11: 13–25.

National Institute of Public Health, Sweden (2004) *Reduced Use of Tobacco – How Far Have We Come?*, Stockholm: National Institute of Public Health, Sweden.

Nazroo, J., Edwards, A. and Brown, G. (1998) 'Gender differences in the prevalence of depression: artefact, alternative disorders, biology or roles?', *Sociology of Health & Illness*, 20 (3): 312–30.

NCHS (National Center for Health Statistics) (2004) *Health, United States, 2004*, Hyattsville, Maryland: National Center for Health Statistics.

Nicholson, L. (1994) 'Interpreting gender', *Signs*, 20: 79–105.

Nicholson, L. (1999) *The Play of Reason. From the Modern to the Postmodern*, Buckingham: Open University Press.

Oakley, A. (1972) *Sex, Gender and Society*, London: Temple Smith.

Oakley, A. (1974a) *The Sociology of Housework*, London: Martin Robertson.

Oakley, A. (1974b) *Housewife*, London: Allen Lane.

Oakley, A. (1975) 'The trap of medicalised motherhood', *New Society*, 18 December: 639–41.

Oakley, A. (1976) 'Wisewoman and Medicine Man: Changes in the Management of Childbirth', in J. Mitchell and A. Oakley (eds) *The Rights and Wrongs of Women*, London: Penguin Books, pp. 17–38.

Oakley, A. (1980) *Women Confined. Towards a Sociology of Childbirth*, New York: Schocken Books.

Oakley, A. (1989) 'Who cares for women? Science versus love in midwifery today', William Power Memorial Lecture, *Midwives Chronicle and Nursing Notes*, July: 214–21.

Oakley, A. (1998) 'A brief history of gender,' in A. Oakley and J. Mitchell (eds) *Who's Afraid of Feminism? Seeing Through the Backlash*, London: Penguin Books, pp. 29–55.

Oakley, A. (2002) *Gender on Planet Earth*, Cambridge: Polity Press.

Oakley, A. (2007) *Fractured. Adventures of a Broken Body*, Bristol: Policy Press.

O'Brien, M. (1981) *The Politics of Reproduction*, London: Routledge/Kegan Paul.

O'Driscoll, K., Stronge, J. M. and Minogue, M. (1972) 'Active management of labour', *British Medical Journal*, 3: 135–7.

Olesen, V. and Whittaker, E. (1968) *The Silent Dialogue. A Study in the Social Psychology of Professional Socialization*, San Francisco, CA: Jossey-Bass.

Olesen, V. and Lewin, E. (1985) 'Women, health, and healing: a theoretical introduction', in E. Lewin and V. Olesen (eds) *Women, Health, and Healing*, London: Tavistock, pp. 1–24.

ONS (Office for National Statistics) (2006a) *Focus on Health*, London: Stationery Office.

ONS (2006b) 'Suicide Rates for men continue to fall', *News Release*, 27 June 2006, available at www/statistics.gov.uk/statbase/product.asp?vink=621.

ONS (2006c) 'Alcohol-related deaths since the 1990s', available at www.statistics. gov.uk/cci/nugget.asp?id=1091 (accessed 11 November 2006).

ONS (2007) *Social Trends 37*, London: Stationery Office.

ONS (2008) *Social Trends 38*, London: Stationery Office.

ONS (n.d.) Derived from ONS Longitudinal Study (Table 1), available at www.statistics.gov.uk.

O'Sullivan, S. (1987) (ed.) *Women's Health. A Spare Rib Reader*, London: Pandora.

Oudshoorn, N. (1994) *Beyond the Natural Body: An Archaeology of Sex Hormones*, London: Routledge.

Pakulski, J. and Waters, M. (1996) *The Death of Class*, London: Sage.

Palmeri, A. (1983) 'Charlotte Perkins Gilman: Forerunner of a feminist social science', in S. Harding and M. B. Hintikka (eds) *Discovering Reality. Feminist Perspectives on Epistemology, Metaphysics, Methodology, and Philosophy of Science*, London: D. Reidel Publishing Company, pp. 97–119.

Pampel, F. (2001) 'Cigarette diffusion and sex differences in smoking', *Journal of Health and Social Behaviour*, 42 (December): 388–404.

Pampel, F. (2002) 'Cigarette use and the narrowing sex differential in mortality', *Population and Development Review*, 28 (1): 77–104.

Pankhurst, C. (1913) *The Great Scourge and How to End It*, London: Lincoln's Inn House.

Parsons, T. (1950) *The Social System*, New York: Free Press.

Parsons, T. and Bales, R. F. (1956) *Family, Socialisation and Interaction Processes*, London: Routledge/Kegan Paul.

Patsopoulos, N., Tatsioni, A. and Ioannidis, J. (2007) 'Claims of sex differences. An empirical assessment in genetic associations', *Journal of the American Medical Association*, 298 (8): 880–93.

Payne, S. (2001) '"Smoke like a man, die like a man?': A review of the relationship between gender, sex and lung cancer', *Social Science & Medicine*, 53 (8): 1067–80.

Payne, S. (2004) 'Sex, gender, and irritable bowel syndrome: making connections', *Gender Medicine*, 1 (1): 18–28.

Payne, S. (2006) *The Health of Men and Women*, Cambridge: Polity Press.

Perenboom, R., van Herten, L., Boshuzien, H. and van den Bos, G. (2005) 'Life expectancy without chronic morbidity: trends in gender and socioeconomic disparities', *Public Health Reports*, 120 (1): 46–54.

Perry, R. (1979) 'The veil of chastity: Mary Astell's feminism', *Studies in Eighteenth Century Culture*, 9: 25–43.

Perry, R. (1986) *The Celebrated Mary Astell*, Chicago, IL: Chicago University Press.

Petersen, S., Peto, V., Scarborough, P. and Rayner, M. (2005) *Coronary Heart Disease Statistics 2005 edition*, London: British Heart Foundation.

Pilcher, J. (1999) *Women in Contemporary Britain*, London: Routledge.

Plechner, D. (2000) 'Women, medicine, and sociology: some thoughts on the need for a critical feminist perspective', in J. Jacobs Kronenfeld (ed.) *Health, Illness and the Use of Care: The Impact of Social Factors*, New York: JAI/Elsevier Science, pp. 69–94.

Poovey, M. (1988) *Uneven Developments. The Ideological Work of Gender in Mid-Victorian England*, Chicago, IL: University of Chicago Press.

Popay, J. and Groves, K. (2000) '"Narrative" in research on gender inequalities in health', in E. Annandale and K. Hunt (eds) *Gender Inequalities in Health*, Buckingham: Open University Press, pp. 64–89.

Pope, H., Phillips, K. and Olivardia, R. (2000) *The Adonis Complex. The Secret Crisis of Male Body Obsession*, New York: Free Press.

Porter, R. (1997) *The Greatest Benefit to Mankind. A Medical History of Humanity from Antiquity to the Present*, London: HarperCollins.

Pringle, R. (1998) *Sex and Medicine: Gender, Power and Authority in the Medical Profession*, Cambridge: Cambridge University Press.

Prokhovnik, R. (1999) *Rational Woman. A Feminist Critique of Dichotomy*, London: Routledge.

Pumphrey, M. (1987) 'The Flapper, the housewife and the making of modernity', *Cultural Studies*, 1 (2): 179–94.

Rapp, R. (2001) 'Gender, body, biomedicine: how some feminist concerns dragged reproduction to the center of social theory', *Medical Anthropology Quarterly*, 15 (4): 466–77.

Rich, A. (1977) *Of Woman Born. Motherhood as Experience and Institution*, London: Virago.

Rich, E. (2005) 'Young women, feminist identities and neo-liberalism', *Women's Studies International Forum*, 28 (6): 495–508.

Riska, E. (2002) 'From type A man to hardy man: masculinity and health', *Sociology of Health & Illness*, 24 (3): 247–358.

Riska, E. (2004) *Masculinity and Men's Health. Coronary Heart Disease in Medical and Public Discourse*, Oxford: Rowman & Littlefield.

Riska, E. and Heikell, T. (2007) 'Gender and images of heart disease in Scandinavian drug advertising', *Scandinavian Journal of Public Health*, 35 (6): 585–90.

Roberts, C. (2002) *The Woman and the Hour. Harriet Martineau and Victorian Ideologies*, London: University of Toronto Press.

Roberts, E. (1995) *Women and Families. An Oral History, 1940–1970*, Oxford: Blackwell.

Robertson, S. (2007) *Understanding Men and Health*, Maidenhead: Open University Press/McGraw Hill.

Rogers, M. F. (1999) *Barbie Culture*, London: Sage.

Roiphe, K. (1993) *The Morning After. Fear and Feminism*, Boston, MA: Little Brown.

Rosen, R. (2000) *The World Spilt Open. How the Modern Women's Movement Changed America*, New York: Viking.

Rosengren, W. and DeVault, S. (1978) 'The sociology of time and space in an obstetrical hospital', in D. Tuckett and J. Kaufert (eds) *Basic Readings in Medical Sociology*, London: Tavistock, pp. 197–203.

Roskies, E. (1978) 'Sex, culture and illness – an overview', *Social Science & Medicine*, 12B: 139–141.

Rossi, A. (1968) 'Transition to parenthood', *Journal of Marriage and the Family*, 30 (1): 26–39.

Rothman, B. K. (1981) 'Awake and aware or false consciousness? The co-optation of childbirth reform in America', in S. Romalis (ed.) *Childbirth: Alternatives to Medical Control*, Austin, TX: University of Texas Press, pp. 150–80.

Rothman, B. K. (1982) *In Labour. Women and Power in the Birth-place*, London: Junction Books.

Rousseau, J. (1966 [1762]) *Émile*, trans. B. Foxley, London: Dent.

Rowbotham, S. (1972) 'The beginnings of women's liberation in Britain', in M. Wandor (ed.) *The Body Politic. Writings from the Women's Liberation Movement in Britain 1969–1972*. London: Stage 1, pp. 91–102.

Rowbotham, S. (1973) *Woman's Consciousness in a Man's World*, London: Pelican Books.

Rowbotham, S. (2000) *Promise of a Dream: Remembering the Sixties*, London: Penguin Books.

Rowe, M. (ed.) (1982) *Spare Rib Reader. 100 Issues of Women's Liberation*, London: Penguin Books.

Rowland, R. and Klein, R. (1996) 'Radical feminism: history, politics, action', in D. Bell and R. Klein (eds) *Radically Speaking. Feminism Reclaimed*, London: Zed Books, pp. 9–36, 37–44.

Rubin, G. (1975) 'The traffic in women: notes on the "political economy" of sex', in R. R. Reiter (ed.) *Toward an Anthropology of Women*, London: Monthly Review Press, pp.157–210.

Ruzek, S. (1978) *The Women's Health Movement: Feminist Alternatives to Medical Control*, London: Praeger.

Ryall, A. (2000) 'Medical body and the lived experience: the case of Harriet Martineau', *Mosaic* (Winnipeg), 33 (4): 35–52.

Ryan, D. (2000) '"All the world and her husband": the Daily Mail Ideal Home Exhibition, 1908–39', in M. Andrews and M. M. Talbot (eds) *All the World and Her Husband. Women in Twentieth-century Consumer Culture*, London: Cassell, pp. 10–22.

Saltonstall, R. (1993) 'Healthy bodies, social bodies: men's and women's concepts and practices of health in everyday life', *Social Science & Medicine* 36 (1): 7–14.

Samet, J. M. and Yoon, S. (2001) *Women and the Tobacco Industry*, Geneva: World Health Organisation.

Sandall, J. (1999) 'Choice, continuity and control: changing midwifery towards a sociological perspective', in E. Van Teijlingen, G. Lowis, P. McCaffery and M. Porter (eds) *Midwifery and the Medicalization of Childbirth. Comparative Perspectives*, New York: Nova Science Publishers, pp. 353–63.

Sandelowski, M. (1981) *Women, Health, and Choice*, Englewood Cliffs, NJ: Prentice-Hall

Sanders, V. (1986) *Reason Over Passion. Harriet Martineau and the Victorian Novel*, Brighton, Sussex: Harvester Press.

Sanders, V. (ed.) (1990) *Harriet Martineau: Selected Letters*, Oxford: Clarendon Press.

Savage, M. (2000) *Class Analysis and Social Transformation*, Buckingham: Open University Press.

Sawicki, J. (1991) *Disciplining Foucault. Feminism, Power and the Body*, London: Routledge.

Scambler, A. (1998) 'Gender, health and the feminist debate on postmodernism', in S. Scambler and P. Higgs (eds) *Modernity, Medicine and Health*, London: Routledge, pp. 100–24.

Scheff, R. (1966) *Being Mentally Ill*, Chicago, IL: Aldine.

Scully, D. (1977) 'Skill-acquisition in obstetrics and gynaecology: social processes and implications for patient care', PhD thesis: University of Illinois.

Scully, D. (1980) *Men Who Control Women's Health*, Boston, MA: Houghton Mifflin.

Scully, D. (2003) 'Afterword', *Feminism and Psychology*, 13 (1): 40–4.

Scully, D. and Bart, P. (1973) 'A funny thing happened on the way to the orifice: women in gynaecology textbooks', *American Journal of Sociology*, 78(4): 1045–51.

Seaman, B. (1995 [1969]) *Doctor's Case Against the Pill*, Alamdea, CA: Hunter House.

Sennett, R. (2006) *The Culture of the New Capitalism*, London: Yale University Press.

Shafey, O., Dolwick, S. and Guindon, G. (2003) *Tobacco Control Country Profiles*, Atlanta, GA: American Cancer Society.

Shapiro, N., Najman, J., Chang, A., Keeping, J., Morrison, J. and Western, J. (1983) 'Information control and the exercise of power in the obstetrical encounter', *Social Science & Medicine*, 17 (3): 139–46.

Shaw, M., Maxwell, R., Rees, K., Davidson, D., Oliver, S., Ben-Shlomo, Y. and Ebrahim, S. (2004) 'Gender and age inequity in the provision of coronary revascularisation in England in the 1990s: is it getting better?', *Social Science & Medicine*, 59 (12): 2499–507.

Shildrick, M. (1997) *Leaky Bodies and Boundaries. Feminism, Postmodernism and (Bio)ethics*, London: Routledge.

Shildrick, M. and Price, J. (1998) 'Introduction', in M. Shildrick and J. Price (eds) *Vital Signs. Feminist Reconfigurations of the Bio/logical Body,* Edinburgh: Edinburgh University Press, pp. 1–17.

Shilling, C. (2003) *The Body and Social Theory,* 2nd edn, London: Sage.

Shilling, C. (2007) 'Sociology and the body: classical traditions and new agendas', in C. Shilling (ed.) *Embodying Sociology: Retrospect, Progress and Prospects,* Oxford: Blackwell/The Sociological Review, pp. 1–18

Shim, J. (2002) 'Understanding the routinised inclusion of race, socioeconomic status and sex in epidemiology: the utility of concepts from technoscience studies', *Sociology of Health & Illness,* 24 (2): 129–50.

Shorter, E. (1982) *A History of Women's Bodies,* London: Penguin Books.

Skeggs, B. (1997) *Formations of Class and Gender,* London: Sage.

Skelton, C., Francis, B. and Valkanova, Y. (2007) *Breaking Down the Stereotypes: Gender and Achievement in Schools,* Manchester: Equal Opportunities Commission.

Smith, D. (1974) 'Women's perspective as a radical critique of sociology', *Sociological Inquiry,* 44: 1–13.

Smith, D. (1978) ' "K is mentally ill". The anatomy of a factual account', *Sociology,* 12 (1): 23–53.

Smith, H. L. (1982) *Reason's Disciples. Seventeenth Century English Feminists,* London: University of Illinois Press.

Smith-Rosenberg, C. (1985) *Disorderly Conduct,* Oxford: Oxford University Press.

Spender, D. (1982) *Women of Ideas. And What Men Have Done to Them,* London: Pandora.

Spivak, G. C. (2006 [1988]) *In Other Worlds,* London: Routledge.

Spring Rice, M. (1939) *Working-class Wives,* London: Pelican Books.

Stacey, J. and Thorne, B. (1985) 'The missing feminist revolution in sociology', *Social Problems,* 32 (4): 301–16.

Stacey, M. (1988) *The Sociology of Health and Healing,* London: Unwin Hyman.

Stanley, L. and Wise, S. (1993) *Breaking out Again,* 2nd edn, London: Routledge.

Stanistreet, D., Bambra, C. and Scott-Samuel, A. (2005) 'Is patriarchy the source of men's higher mortality?', *Journal of Epidemiology and Community Health,* 59 (10): 873–6.

Statistics Canada (2001) 'Death – shifting trends', *Health Reports,* 12 (3): 41–6.

Stephens, L. (2004) 'Pregnancy', in M. Stewart (ed.) *Pregnancy, Birth and Maternity Care. Feminist Perspectives,* London: Books for Midwives, pp. 41–56.

Stoller, R. (1968) *Sex and Gender,* New York: Science House.

Strong, P. (1979) 'Sociological imperialism and the profession of medicine: a critical examination of the thesis of medical imperialism', *Social Science & Medicine,* 13a: 199–215.

Sullivan, D. and Weitz, R. (1988) *Labour Pains. Modern Midwives and Home Birth,* London: Yale University Press.

Sundquist, K., Theobald, H., Yang, M., Li, X., Johansson, S. and Sundquist, J. (2006) 'Neighbourhood violent crime and unemployment increase the risk of coronary heart disease: a multilevel study in an urban setting', *Social Science & Medicine,* 62 (8): 2061–71.

Swedish Match (2007) website available at www.swedishmatch.com/eng/Search. asp?q=women (accessed 19 February 2007).

Symonds, A. and Hunt, S. (1996) *The Midwife and Society*, London: Palgrave Macmillan.

Taylor, M. (2000) 'Is midwifery dying?' *Midwifery Matters*, 84 (Spring), available at www.radmid.demon.co.uk/megtaylor.htm (accessed 29 September 2004).

Tew, M. (1990) *Safer Childbirth? A Critical History of Maternity Care*, London: Chapman & Hall.

Thane, P. (1994) 'Women since 1945', in P. Johnson (ed.) *Twentieth-century Britain*, Harlow, Essex: Longman, pp. 392–410.

Thorne, B. (1997) 'Brandeis as a generative institution: critical perspectives, marginality, and feminism', in B. Laslett and B. Thorne (eds) *Feminist Sociology. Life Histories of a Movement*, New Brunswick, NJ: Rutgers University Press, pp. 103–25.

Tocqueville, A. de (1967 [1835,1840]) *Democracy in America*, New York: Harper & Row.

Toll, B. A. and Ling, P, M. (2005) 'The Virginia Slims identity crisis: an inside look at tobacco industry marketing to women', *Tobacco Control*, 14: 172–80.

Tong, R. (1998) *Feminist Thought*, 2nd edn, Oxford: Westview Press.

Tong, R. (2007) 'Feminist thought in transition: never a dull moment', *The Social Science Journal*, 44 (1): 23–39.

Touraine, A. (1998) 'Sociology without society', *Current Sociology*, 46 (2): 119–43.

Trego, L. (2005) 'The integration of feminism and midwifery', *Journal of Midwifery and Women's Health*, 50 (3), 257–8.

Treichler, P. A. (1990) 'Feminism, medicine, and the meaning of childbirth', in M. Jacobus, E. Fox Keller and S. Shuttleworth (eds) *Body/politics*, London: Routledge, pp. 113–38.

Tsuchiya, A. and Williams, A. (2004) 'A "fair innings" between the sexes: are men being treated equally?', *Social Science & Medicine*, 60 (2): 277–86.

Turner, B. (1996) *The Body and Society*, 2nd edn, London: Sage.

Turner, C. (1969) *Family and Kinship in Modern Britain*, London: Routledge & Kegan Paul.

UNESCO (United Nations Educational, Scientific and Cultural Organisation) (2003) *UNESCO's Gender Mainstreaming Implementation Framework for 2002–2000*, Paris: Bureau of Strategic Planning – Section for Women and Gender Equality.

Unal, B., Critchley, J. and Capewell, S. (2004) 'Explaining the decline in coronary heart disease mortality in England and Wales between 1981 and 2000', *Circulation*, 9 March: 1101–7.

Urla, J. and Swedlund, A. C. (1995) 'The anthropometry of Barbie: unsettling ideals of the feminine body in popular culture', in J. Terry and J. Urla (eds) *Deviant Bodies*, Bloomington, IN: University of Indiana Press, pp. 277–313.

Urry, J. (2003) *Global Complexity*, Cambridge: Polity Press.

Vallin, J., Meslé, F. and Valkonen, T. (2001) *Trends in Mortality and Differential Mortality*, Strasbourg: Council of Europe Publishing.

Verbrugge, L. (1983) 'Multiple roles and the physical health of men and women', *Journal of Health and Social Behavior*, 24 (March): 6–30.

Verbrugge, L. (1985) 'Gender and health: an update on hypotheses and evidence', *Journal of Health and Social Behavior,* 26 (September): 156–82.

Verbrugge, L. (1988) 'Unveiling higher morbidity for men. The story', in M. White Riley (ed.) *Social Structures and Human Lives*, London: Sage, pp. 138–60.

Vineis, P., Alavanja, M., Buffler, P., Fontham, E., Franceschi, S., Gao, Y. T., Gupta, P. C., Hackshaw, A., Matos, E., Samet, J., Sitas, F., Smith, J., Stayner, L., Straif, K., Thun, M. J., Wichmann, H. E., Wu, A. H., Zaridze, D., Peto, R. and Doll, R. (2004) 'Tobacco and cancer: recent epidemiological evidence', *Journal of the National Cancer Institute*, 96: 99–106.

Vogel, L. (1995) *Woman Questions. Essays For a Materialist Feminism*, London: Pluto Press.

Wajcman, J. (1991) *Feminism Confronts Technology*, Cambridge: Polity Press.

Wajcman, J. (2004) *Techno Feminism*, Cambridge: Polity Press.

Walby, S. (1997) *Gender Transformations*, London: Routledge.

Walby, S. (2007) *Gender (In)equality and the Future of Work*, London: Equal Opportunities Commission.

Waldron, I. (1976) 'Why do women live longer than men?', *Social Science & Medicine*, 10: 349–62.

Waldron, I. (1983a) 'Sex differences in human mortality: the role of genetic factors', *Social Science & Medicine*, 17 (6): 321–33.

Waldron, I. (1983b) 'Sex differences in illness incidence, prognosis and mortality: issues and evidence', *Social Science & Medicine*, 17 (16): 1107–23.

Waldron, I. (1993) 'Recent trends in sex mortality ratios for adults in developed countries', *Social Science & Medicine*, 36 (4): 451–62.

Waldron, I. (2000) 'Trends in gender differences in mortality: relationships to changing gender differences in behaviour and other causal factors', in E. Annandale and K. Hunt (eds) *Gender Inequalities in Health*, Buckingham: Open University Press, pp. 150–81.

Waldron, I., Weiss, C. and Hughes, E. (1989) 'Interacting effects of multiple roles on women's health', *Journal of Health and Social Behavior*, 39: 216–36.

Walkerdine, V., Lucey, H. and Melody, J. (2001) *Growing Up Girl. Psychosocial Explorations of Gender and Class*, London: Palgrave.

Walkowitz, J. R. (1980) *Prostitution and Victorian Women: Women, Class and the State*, Cambridge: Cambridge University Press.

Wallen, J., Waitzkin, H. and Stoeckle, J. (1979) 'Physician stereotypes about female health and illness: a study of patient's sex and the informative process during medical interviews', *Women and Health*, 4 (2): 135–46.

Walsh, D. (2004) 'Feminism and intrapartum care: a quest for holistic birth', in M. Stewart (ed.) *Pregnancy, Birth and Maternity Care. Feminist Perspectives*, London: Books for Midwives, pp. 57–70.

Waterson, J. (2000) *Women and Alcohol in Context. Mother's Ruin Revisited*, London: Palgrave.

Weber, M. (1949) *The Methodology of the Social Sciences,* trans. and ed. E. A. Shils and H. A. Finch, New York: Free Press.

Weedon, C. (1999) *Feminism, Theory and the Politics of Difference*, Oxford: Blackwell.

Weisman, C. (1998) *Women's Health Care: Activist Traditions and Institutional Change*, Baltimore, MD: Johns Hopkins University Press.

Whelehan, I. (2000) *Overloaded. Popular Culture and the Future of Feminism*, London: The Women's Press.

White, A. and Cash, K. (2004) 'The state of men's health in Europe', *Journal of Men's Health and Gender*, 1 (1): 60–6.

White, A. and Holmes, M. (2006) 'Patterns of mortality across 44 countries among men and women aged 15–44 years, *Journal of Men's Health and Gender*, 3 (2): 139–51.

White, C., van Glen, F. and Chow, Y. (2003) 'Trends in social class differences in mortality by cause, 1986 to 2000', *Health Statistics Quarterly*, 20 (Winter): 25–37.

Whitehead, S. (2002) *Men and Masculinities. Key Themes and New Directions*, Cambridge: Polity Press.

WHO (World Health Organisation) (2001) *Mainstreaming Gender Equity in Health: The Need to Move Forward*, Copenhagen: WHO Regional Office for Europe.

Williams, S. (2003) *Medicine and the Body*, London: Sage.

Williams, S. and Bendelow, G. (1998) *The Lived Body*, London: Routledge.

Wilson, R. (1970) *The Sociology of Health: An Introduction*, New York: Random House.

Wiltshire, J. (1997) *Jane Austen and the Body. The Picture of Health*, London: Cambridge University Press.

Winter, A. (1998) *Mesmerized. Powers of Mind in Victorian Britain*, London: University of Chicago Press.

Wise, S. and Stanley, L. (2003) 'Review. Looking back and looking forward: some recent feminist sociology reviewed', *Sociological Research Online*, 8 (3), available at www.socresonline.org.uk/8/3/wise.html.

Wizemann, T. M. and Pardue, M. (2001) *Exploring the Biological Contributions to Human Health. Does Sex Matter?*, Washington, DC: National Academy Press.

Wolf, A. (2006) 'Working girls', *Prospect Magazine*, 121 (April), www.prospect-magazine.co.uk/article_details.php?id=7398 (accessed 25 April 2006).

Wolf, N. (1994) *Fire with Fire*, London: Virago.

Wollstonecraft, M. (1992 [1792]) *A Vindication of the Rights of Woman*, London: Penguin Books.

Wood, J. (2001) *Passion and Pathology in Victorian Fiction*, London: Oxford University Press.

Woodham-Smith, C. (1950) *Florence Nightingale 1820–1910*, London: Constable.

Wright Mills, C. (1975 [1959]) *The Sociological Imagination*, Harmondsworth: Penguin Books.

Young, I. (1981) 'Beyond the unhappy marriage: a critique of dual systems theory', in Lydia Sargent (ed.) *Women and Revolution*, London: Pluto Press, pp. 44–69.

Young, I. (2005) 'Introduction', in I. Young, *On Female Body Experience*, Oxford: Oxford University Press, pp. 3–11.

Yuen, P. (2005) *Compendium of Health Statistics 2005–2006*, London: Office of Health Economics.

Zailckas, K. (2005) *Smashed. Growing Up a Drunk Girl*, London: Ebury Press.

Zalewski, K. (1990) 'Logical contradictions in feminist health care: a rejoinder to Peggy Foster', *Journal of Social Policy*, 19: 235–44.

Zalewski, M. (2000) *Feminism After Postmodernism. Theorising Through Practice*, London: Routledge.

Zweniger-Bargielowska, I. (2001a) 'Housewifery', in I. Zweniger-Bargielowska (ed.) *Women in Twentieth-century Britain*, London: Longman, pp. 149–64.

Zweniger-Bargielowska, I. (2001b) 'Introduction', in I. Zweniger-Bargielowska (ed.) *Women in Twentieth-century Britain*, London: Longman, pp. 1–15.

Index